Hip Replacement or Hip Resurfacing

A Story of Choices

By

Peggy Gabriel

ISBN: 1-4107-6566-0 (e-book)
ISBN: 1-4107-6565-2 (Paperback)

This book is printed on acid free paper.

1stBooks - rev. 08/20/03

Table Of Contents

* * *

Section One
The Path of Discovery

Section Two
Resurfacing: The Bone-Saving Technique

Nineteen
Week sixteen and my well overflows!

Section Three
Cases And Experiences

Disclaimer

If you are about to make decisions to have surgery or treatment I strongly advise that you consult with an experienced physician. My hope is that these pages will be of assistance to you in formulating the questions that you ask your doctor.

I am not a doctor. I do not represent any of the manufacturers, products, or surgeons mentioned in this book.

My viewpoints, and the viewpoints of others expressed in this book, are to be considered as aids, and not catalysts in the understanding of the reader.

Peg Gabriel

Acknowledgments

With the help and encouragement of the following people, the hopes to help others with this book have been made possible. My gratitude flows abundantly to Dr. Koen De Smet, Audrey Ellzey, the people involved with the Surfacehippy Discussion Board, the people involved with the Totallyhip Discussion Board, D'Jango Sanders, Ruth Galinis, Dr. Kelly Coogan, Tricia Coogan, Jillian Coogan, Camille Thomason, Charlie West, Marge Henry, my friends at Office Depot in Corpus Christi, Texas, Vasu Mistry, and my dog, Lulu.

Introduction
By Dr. Koen De Smet

My observances of the suffering and misfortunes of others around me were a determining factor for my decision to specialize in joint surgery. When I became aware of the Hip Resurfacing procedure, I knew that it was to become a part of my practice, as it was definitely the most sensible method for my younger and more active patients. The bone saving qualities and big ball effect of Hip Resurfacing affords to patients the ability to participate in their life activities without the limitations that a typical total hip replacement may present.

The metal on metal technique, <u>without polyethylene</u>, that I use today on my patients, is completely different from the method that I had originally learned. The posterolateral approach (from behind), is part of the formula for success in the surgeries I perform. Important muscles are not cut with this method and healing is more rapid.

Many of my patients who were deemed ineligible for Resurfacing by other physicians now enjoy the fruits of a Birmingham Hip Resurfacing (BHR) surgery. It is my privilege to allow candidates the choice between total hip replacement and a BHR. For this reason I remained at the University of Ghent. My gratitude expands to see my patients plan an active life that is free from pain. This is why I love my work.

When I first became involved with the Resurfacing technique, I did not realize that I would become instrumental in spreading the knowledge of this to many parts of the world. Not only do I speak in different parts of the globe, but patients come to me for the BHR from many countries. My hopes for the future for this technique is that surgeons will be well educated in the procedure, that the other Resurfacing prostheses coming on the market will have a good metallurgy, and lastly, that the other good products that are now on the market, are not discontinued for the sake of financial gain. I foresee that someday as research brings us new knowledge, physicians will have new and better ways to help their patients.

The bridges between the medical profession and its patients can be huge. The personal stories of this book may prove to be very beneficial to the average person who does not find accessibility to medical journals or the internet an easy endeavor. The experiences and knowledge shared in this book may or may not be that of my own patients. It does not matter. The bringing of clarity about a very beneficial surgical procedure to the many who are searching for answers is what I wish to promote.

Preface

More than 800,000 artificial hip joints have been implanted in the U.S. *1* A very high percentage of these surgeries have been performed on people who are over fifty years of age. The baby boomers are now reaching a time when hip joint replacement can become a reality in their lives. The number of hip replacement surgeries performed each year is constantly rising. It is estimated that the number of hip replacements performed in the United States annually has risen to 120,000. *2*

The events described in this book reflect the challenges and victories of many who searched for and found the gift of choice. Choice, the self-given prize, is the wisdom to learn about alternatives. This story touches pain in a very true sense: the pain of losing something and the quest to get it back. In sharing this information, the writer hopes that the reader will find the acknowledgment of the blessing of being able to live life in a normal way and participate in the joys, of which we all are deserving. Some of the names have been changed, but every character is a real person, who had to deal with doctors, ignorance, fear, humiliation, pain, and often insurance companies.

This book offers information to those facing hip surgery. Many people are still not informed of all of the available options. Due to the lack of information, the choice of Hip Resurfacing creates fear in many. Being able to learn from the experience and research of others, as well as my own, has proven to be far more valuable than just accepting the answers that were given to me from educated persons in the medical field, for they too, are still learning. What I learned from first hand experience is that a physician may not be aware of all of the ever-changing options that we have. From personal experience in seeking answers, it is clear that we should use our doctors' knowledge as a tool, and be open constantly for more information from other sources. The world keeps changing in leaps and bounds before our eyes. New technology is pouncing upon us constantly, and we need to become knowledgeable about new possibilities before we judge and reject them.

Although this book often refers to my own Belgium surgery experience, it is definitely representative to such a surgery done anywhere. The information that this book offers is from different parts of the world, as this procedure expands across our globe.

Those who are facing the possibility of having a total hip replacement (THR), or know of someone who is considering such an operation, should read this book. My hope is to create an understanding about hip surgery and the options that are there for us. Peg Gabriel

SECTION ONE

THE PATH OF DISCOVERY

One

You'll Never Miss the Water 'til the Well Runs Dry

The cool mountain air filled my lungs as I hiked up the trail in beautiful Big Bend National Park in West Texas. Something different from the norm nagged for my attention. I was not keeping up with my family. They were ahead of me and I found that I was struggling to match their gait. It had been a year since we last hiked together, on our vacation in Colorado. Even then, I remembered that I was weaker in my pace, experiencing a dull pain that caused me to sit and rest at intervals on long hikes.

I was in my mid forties and appeared to be fit. Finding pride in my ability to walk fast with long strides seemed to be a thing of the past. Recognizing that I seemed to have lost a great deal of strength in my legs, brought me some concerns. This was to mark the beginning of another kind of trail for me, abundant with undeniable signs that would eventually lead to a life-changing decision.

My life otherwise seemed normal. I rode horses, fetched kids, shagged balls at softball practices, and walked a mile every day. All of the time, there was a nagging pain that seemed to come from my lower back. I was once told by a doctor that I had a bone spur on L5. I often thought that this was the cause of the pain. If I stood for any length of time, or walked a long distance, that pain would always become more intense. I learned to live with it. I ignored it unless it screamed for some relief from over the counter painkillers.

As time went on, my lower back pain affected my life. I found that I cleaned house less efficiently. Dreading to stand in long lines at stores led me to avoid shopping for food, clothing, and even Christmas gifts as much as possible. If I had to stand at a church service, I would leave. Everybody seems to stand at parties, sharing conversations. I found this to be a painful experience. I learned to do a squat to relieve the pressure in my lower back. If I was out in

3

public, and the needed squat would draw too much attention, I would invent a reason to stoop to pick up something from the ground and use that fleeting moment to affect the needed stretch in my lower back and alleviate the pain. I had seen a couple of chiropractors who treated my back. One even put me into arch supports, which I am sure that I needed. But not one of them saw what was going on in my hips.

My neck began to participate in the dance of pain. It hurt all of the time. I went to other physicians. The problem in my spine was always recognized, and efforts to relax the muscle tension along with other therapies were exercised. I was told that the lower back problem was a connection to the neck pain.

The temporary solutions seemed more futile when my back became inflamed while I was working on a difficult yoga posture. I had this pain before, and felt I could manage it. When it did not get better, I went to my doctor and had MRIs. I was told that I had a spondylolisthesis at L5, which is a vertebrae that moves outward like a shelf. This was not an uncommon condition, as it was explained to me. It is a condition that many people have and some are not even aware of it. The degree of my spondylolisthesis was not anything serious. I was given some physical therapy exercises to do. The physical therapy felt nice, but as soon as I walked the pain returned without mercy. By that time, walking was so burdensome that I avoided it as much as I could. Gratefully, I could do my Pilates exercises. I had been teaching a Pilates exercise mat work routine at a local gym as well as in my private studio. Laying on the mat without the pressure from standing, allowed me to demonstrate the exercises. Lower back stretches with the knee brought to the chest really seemed to be an important part of my pain management, and this was a repetitive movement in the Pilates routine that I taught.

To be able to walk and not think about it is a gift. The old adage, "you never miss the water until the well runs dry" came to mind when appreciating the ability to walk. With time, matters worsened. If I had to cross a street, I needed to make sure that there were not any cars coming, as I could not hasten my step, or trot, if necessary to avoid being hit. One day, while I was crossing a busy street, a speeding car came unexpectedly from around a curve. Being unable to run, I stood petrified in fear. I knew that I would not make it to safety on time no matter how much effort was exerted. I closed my eyes and waited to be struck down. The car swerved around me, honking his horn angrily. My feelings of being intimidated by traffic began to influence my walks.

Assessing the degree of success of each of my walks by how many times I had to rest became the norm. My right leg was longer than my left. A chiropractor thought that perhaps heel lifts would make them the same length and decrease pain. If it did decrease the pain, it was not by much.

I managed through another year of creative pain avoidance. By this time, it seemed that all facets of my life were tainted with pain. As I gave up dancing and nature hikes, I became interested in kayaking. With the assistance of friends, who would do most of the carrying, I could get out into nature to see the birds and wildlife.

With ever increasing problems, again I went to my doctor. X-rays and MRIs were ordered. I dreaded what they would say. I felt strongly that it would reveal a need for some serious spinal surgery. Having friends who have had spinal surgery, and who will probably live in pain for the rest of their lives, I knew that there were risks involved. The tests revealed that the problem in my back had worsened. Another doctor recommended physical therapy for my back, which was futile, for as soon as I walked, the pain returned without mercy. An appointment was made for me to see a specialist in a neighboring city. He told me that this doctor was one of the best for the evaluation that I needed.

Two

Spinal problems and Hip problems

With my MRIs in hand, I limped up to the office of the specialist. My fear was probably easily detected in my words and voice. He seemed very compassionate as he made queries about my pain. He spoke about spinal fusions and reassured me on how frequently these surgeries take place with success.

As I searched for clarity, his answers brought me to a state of doubt. If I were to allow this fusion, it could effect the next vertebrae, and another fusion could be needed later. My yoga and Pilates would be more limited with one fusion, yet with two, and would there be three?

The doctor appeared astonished when he finally looked at my X-rays. He interjected into the conversation the most shocking information. I was also in need of hip surgery. By showing me my X-rays, he helped me to see that my left hip was bone on bone and the right hip had very little cartilage left. He reassured me that I would be fine and that I would be able to remain active. He never did tell me about the limitations I would face after receiving a total hip replacement. He set an appointment for my surgery, which was for a double hip replacement as well as a spinal fusion. My insurance was going to cover the majority of the costs and everything seemed to be a "go."

Was I on the path that I wanted to be on? My mind would not let me rest. During the drive home, I made a pact with myself that I would cancel the surgery until I knew more about the procedures as well as the physicians available. A second opinion would also be in order.

The next morning, I was wakened early because my old dog was whining. She could not get up because her hips were jaded from age. She had dysplasia. While peering at the reflection in the mirror of my nude hips, I felt depressed. I was only 51 years old, very active, and now discovering that I had tattered, threadbare, and dilapidated hips.

I truly matched my dog. "That's what they say, isn't it?" I thought. "A dog often reflects its master, taking on the demeanor or certain traits of its human." It hurt as I bent over to feed my dog. I felt bitter that I had to face the possibility of having a spinal fusion surgery as well as having two hips replaced. With the hope that perhaps it was not true, I had my doctor refer me to a spinal specialist. I told him that I wanted an experienced spinal man to whom he would send his own wife. An appointment was set up.

That afternoon, I went onto the Internet and began typing in searches. I discovered that I could find out specific things about doctors with great ease. I typed in a search for spinal surgery. An abundance of information came up onto my computer screen, including names of doctors. When I looked up the doctor that I had an appointment with, I discovered that his number one specialty was not the spine, nor the hips. His first specialty was tumors. Actually, the spine was listed sixth in his specialties. Not doubting for a moment that it would be best to go to a doctor who specialized in the spine first, I researched until I found one who impressed me. This specialist was in Houston. He not only invented implants for the spine, but he also spoke around the world about his specialty. With ease, I made an appointment, with a simple phone call and some insurance information. I did not need to have a referral from my doctor. I was told to bring my tests.

Three

It's the Hips, not the Spine!

As I walked into the clinic for my appointment with the spinal specialist, I tried not to limp. I did my squat for a several seconds, to alleviate the lower back pain. The wait to see the doctor was not a lengthy one.

The doctor evaluated my X-rays and MRIs, as well as my gait. He seemed to be quite thorough. "I would never operate on your spine," he began. The doctor gained my trust when he explained that he believed that the spondylolisthesis condition in my spine was common and even seen in athletes. He added that one could live with this condition and be free from pain with proper management. Bringing me to the reality that the deterioration of my hips, and the manner in which I was being forced to walk from that condition, was harming my lower back, he added, "If you fix the hips, more than likely your spine will straighten itself out, and very likely you will see a great improvement in your neck." With reassurance, he added that if problems were to continue after the hips were repaired, I could always return to him for further evaluation. His evaluation of my situation was that it was most likely hereditary, and that something needed to be done about it soon for the sake of the spine.

Now I understood why I found that the pilates mat work to be far easier than the act of walking. Laying on a Pilates mat, without any weight on my hips and spine, and doing the routine proved to be extremely valuable for the muscles in every part of my body, while not putting weight on my hips. While this fact was true, ironically, the very act of walking was an enemy to my spine. Elated with gratitude that I did not need to go through with the spinal surgery, the need to see a hip replacement specialist was evident.

A good friend of mine happened to work for a very well thought of hip replacement specialist in South Texas. She made the appointment for me immediately.

As the hip replacement specialist viewed my X-rays, he seemed to be very matter of fact. The degeneration of my left hip was advancing. He explained that it was bone on bone. Like the other doctor, he concurred that the right hip was well on its way to serious degeneration and the cartilage was almost gone.

The doctors' honesty of how my life would change from this surgery was very painful, but valuable. No longer would I teach my fitness classes. Bringing the knees to the chest, crossing the legs, and various movements that were required of me as a Pilates teacher could cause a dislocation. I probed with questions to find other solutions, and the doctor had none.

In an obvious attempt to show me brighter possibilities, he reported to me the activities that his other patients enjoyed: swimming, bicycle riding, power walking, golf, and dancing. With a wave of sorrow swelling up inside of me, yet remaining outwardly calm enough to maintain some aspect of composure, I asked about kayaking. He asked me to imitate how I got into my boat. As I demonstrated the motion to him, the answer was "sell the kayak." The seriousness of dislocation would always have to be considered with two artificial hips.

In knowing that this all meant I would never be able to do the low back spine stretches that relieved my back pain I wondered how I could manage if the back pain continued after the hip surgery. I knew I would not be able to squat and pee in the woods anymore. Sitting on a low log around a campfire would not be in my life. Sitting on the floor would have to be done with great care and probably not at all. If I went camping, I would have to consider all of these factors. He said that the double total hip replacement would give me about eight to twelve years on each hip, at best, before a revision surgery would be required. After that, I would be on a cycle of such revision surgeries for the rest of my life. I found myself in mourning.

My insurance company responded that they would pay their part for this hip replacement surgery, and a date was set. I walked out of his office feeling like I was having a bad dream.

Reflections on the doctor's words about the hereditary factor caused me to wonder if my children would be prone to this. My parents did not have any hip problems, but the problem did peek out its ugly head with my aunt and my grandmother.

This triggered memories of my grandmother and caused me to feel ever closer to her, as after all, I inherited a condition that she had. When I was younger, I shared wondrous walks with my grandmother around her huge flower garden. She had acres of flowers and would tell me about each and every type that she grew. The joy she expressed when she told me the stories that her mother had told her about the flowers, made the colors and fragrances even more breathtaking. Slowly, her garden dwindled. Over a period of several years, her garden became progressively smaller and more neglected, until her flower tending was reduced to a potted plant on the back porch. The ever-increasing pain in her hips had been robbing her of the fortitude to work in the garden. I watched this diva of the flowers transform into a chair-ridden woman. She was told by her doctor to wait as long as possible before she went under the knife for a total hip replacement. Finally, at eighty-four years of age, the decision was made that it was time for the surgery.

I was there the day after her hip replacement surgery, when they were getting her up to walk for the first time. I will never forget the words she spoke when she first was assisted into a standing position. She stood with her elderly body and a surgical procedure leaving a long scar, muscles cut, stitches and bruising. Her words were, "It feels better now." To have said that, in my view, decreed how horrendous her pain must have been before the surgery. She never did return to her gardening. I often think of what a pity it was that she was forced to wait for so long to get the surgery. To miss out on even a year of life because of pain is a shame.

Four

Meet The Hipsters

The next morning, I went onto the Internet to learn more about hip replacement surgery. There was an easily found site called the Totally Hip Discussion Board. The posts were abundant from many people who had already received a total hip replacement, as well as from people who were considering the surgery. Those who already had a total hip replacement called themselves "Hipsters". With a strange sort of eagerness, laced with hesitation, I began to read about the pros, cons, and facts about hip degeneration and the total hip replacement (THR).

With ever increasing clarity, I knew there were many things that a doctor might not tell me unless I asked, if I knew what to ask, that could be found on this Board. The Hipsters seemed to delve into everything. Some of the posts were quite disturbing, including stories about dislocations, fractures, infections, pain, and revisions. There were some descriptions of how the long part of the prosthesis, which is inserted into the hollowed out marrow of the femur, can be the cause of pain in the quads in many people after surgery. Some of the Hipsters spoke of a dropped foot, which resulted from nerve damage during their surgery. The pros and cons of this surgery were not hidden from anyone reading these posts. The Hipsters were generous in sharing their experiences. Every question that I posted received at least one answer if not many.

Facts that did not mean anything to me one mere month before were now vitally important. For instance, information about failure rates with this particular surgery brought me to a new reality. Of course there had to be a failure rate. As one would expect, as with many surgical procedures, there is always a percentage of failures or problems. There is a small, but definite, failure rate for total hip replacements in the United States. 3

What does failure mean in a total hip replacement? There were plenty of posts on this subject to give one a better understanding. The failures that were mentioned were caused from brittle bones, fractures, infections, dislocations, and various other factors. Even though the possibility of failure is upsetting, one has to remember the purpose of the procedure, which is not to create the negative, but to help the patient. There were many more positive stories than negative. It is our responsibility to consider every possibility when facing such a major surgery. Before we leap, we need to have a complete understanding and be accepting of the risks we are taking. The choices we make will be ours to live with.

While checking out more of the details, I learned that the danger of infection with a hip implant is also something that a patient will always have to remain on guard about. The fact is, a bacterial infection can present danger to the artificial joint because the infection could seed in the joint and create the need for surgery. Such surgery could entail removal of the artificial joint with no replacement until the infection is eradicated. Dental work, or any procedure that could produce such an infection, needs to be preceded by an antibiotic treatment to prevent such a nightmare. After THR surgery, it is necessary to always be aware of what is going on in your body, for the sake of preventing such infections as well as other problems that could arise.

Revisions were the outstanding hardship for the Hipsters on the Board. Surgery to revise is always expected. On the posts, it was mentioned that some athletes burn through their Total Hip Replacement in as little as two to five years and have increased dislocation rates. The normal time span for revision seemed to be an average of ten years. Every time a revision is done, more bone is lost, thus the possibility exists of running out of sufficient bone in the future after multiple surgeries. With each revision, the recovery time is longer. For me, I found it to be far easier to accept the life changing limitations that I would experience as a result of this surgery than the idea of foregoing revisions. I felt the need to learn more about the revision experience.

When addressing the question to the Board about what would happen after several revisions, in which bone would be lost each time, I was told that there would be a possibility of ending up in a wheelchair. This is why many people are told to hang on to their own hips and bear the pain as long as possible.

On the Totallyhip Board, one could find it very difficult to feel self-pity for long. There were many who had problems far worse than mine. There were a few under thirty who had to have this surgery. There was one child that was spoken of, who was only ten. There were stories of having many joints replaced, severe arthritis, wheelchairs, and great pain. This surgery improved the quality of life for many.

Regardless of the encouraging stories by the Hipsters, I still felt strongly about wanting to preserve as much of my life as I could. My decision depended on a little more research, yet I needed to decide with some urgency, some education, and some prayer. If only there were another solution. I truly felt fearful of how a double Total Hip Replacement would change my life. What choice did I have? Was there some other way? I was too young to be thinking of having perhaps three or more revision operations for both hips in my lifetime, along with the recuperating time. Even though it is a Godsend for some, and perhaps for myself also, I was not happy with it. If there were only a way to at least buy some time, perhaps ten years, so I could continue my Pilates and yoga. If only there was some other answer.

How ungrateful could I be? If this were fifty years ago, I would end up on the front porch in a rocking chair playing the fiddle like a crippled lady that I used to know. I momentarily conceded to the fact that I would just have to accept this. To blend with it like a chameleon would, as humans are so good at adapting. But still, something kept on nagging at me to check it out even more before I took the big leap.

Five

The Total Hip Replacement

With the Total Hip Replacement operation, the femoral head and neck are removed. Some people may call that the ball of the hip. The marrow space of the femoral canal is reamed out to create space for a metal stem, which has a ball on the end. The metal ball is to replace the amputated bone. Sometimes they use a bone cement, or they may press fit. The idea is to have the bone grow into it. A cup, which may be lined with a polyethylene surface, is set into the pelvis.

The wearing of the polyethylene surface can cause debris from wear, potentially causing bone loss. This bone loss is called Osteolysis. [4] It can cause the implant to loosen, thus the need for revision surgery.

I read about the Polyethylene hazards on ActiveJoints.com, as well as on the Board. I felt that I would want to avoid having any Polyethylene put into my body.

The metal on metal hip replacement is made of cobalt and chromium. The hardness of the metal creates a great reduction in wearing and debris. With this knowledge, I felt that a metal on metal hip replacement was superior to the others. Metal on metal implants have been used in Europe for over twenty years. [5] They are made by Wright Medical, Sulzer (Metasul), and Biomet. They are being marketed under FDA approval in the United States. On the Totally Hip discussion Board, there was a great deal of discussion about different types of hip replacement prosthetics and one could gather numerous opinions. Being shown where to go on the Internet to read about the implant devices was enlightening. It was amazing for me to learn that there are more than sixty different types of hip prosthetics manufactured by nineteen different companies. All of them have the long metal stem to be inserted into the femoral canal after the amputation of the head of the femur (the ball of the hip).

Diagrams Of The Total Hip Replacement

Figure 1.

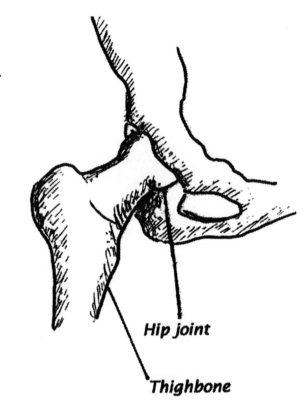

Hip joint

Thighbone

Figure 2.

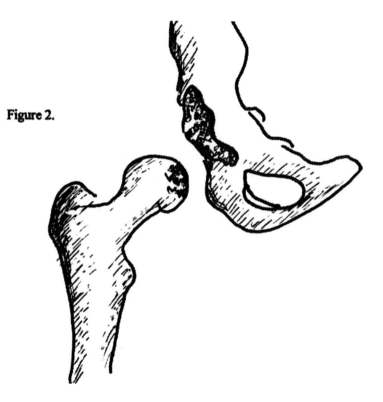

The thighbone is separated from the hip socket

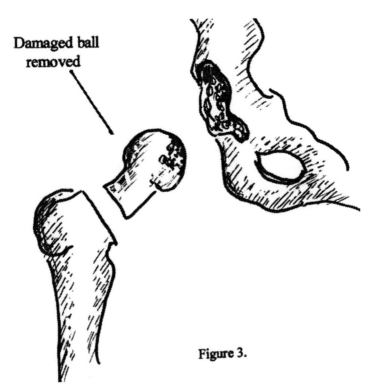

Damaged ball
removed

Figure 3.

The damaged ball is amputated from the thighbone

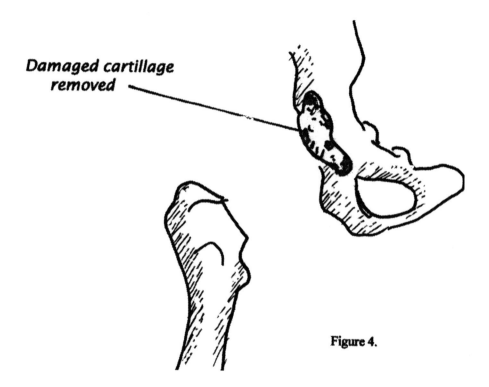

**Damaged cartillage
removed**

Figure 4.

Metal shell

Figure 5.

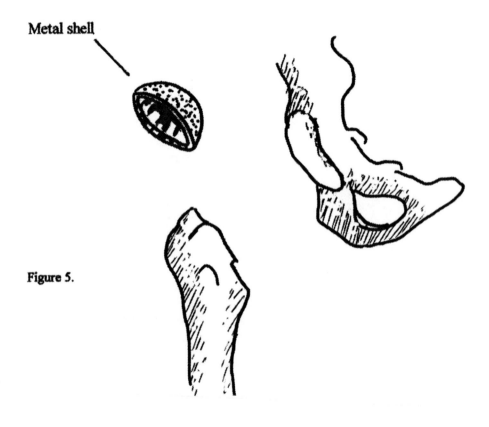

A metal shell is pressed into the socket of the hip

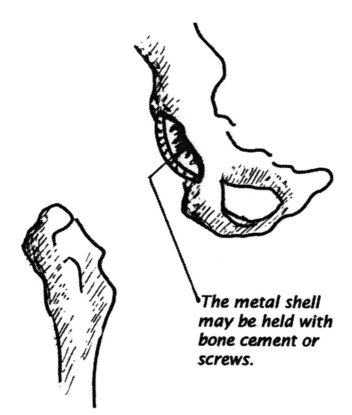

The metal shell may be held with bone cement or screws.

Figure 6.

To complete the artificial hip socket, a special liner, which is made of plastic, is secured into the metal shell.

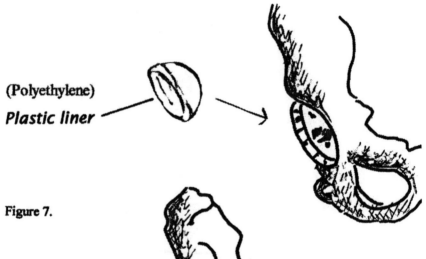

(Polyethylene)

Plastic liner

Figure 7.

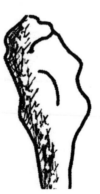

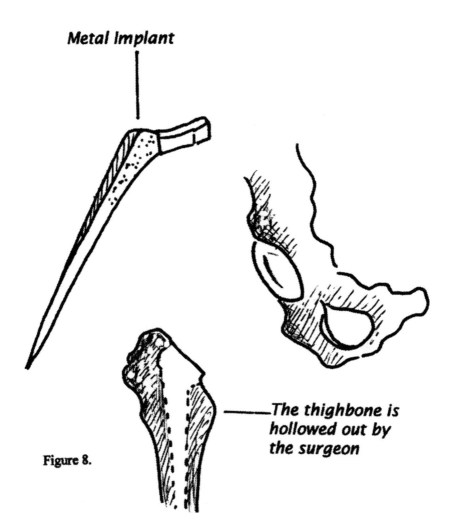

Metal Implant

The thighbone is hollowed out by the surgeon

Figure 8.

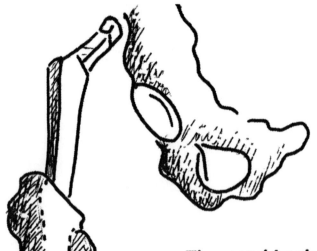

The metal implant is
Carefully placed into
The top of the thigh bone.
Depending on the situation,
Cement may, or may not
Be used.

Figure 9.

24

A ball which is made of Metal or ceramic, is put Onto the stem.   It will Imitate the original ball.

Metal ball

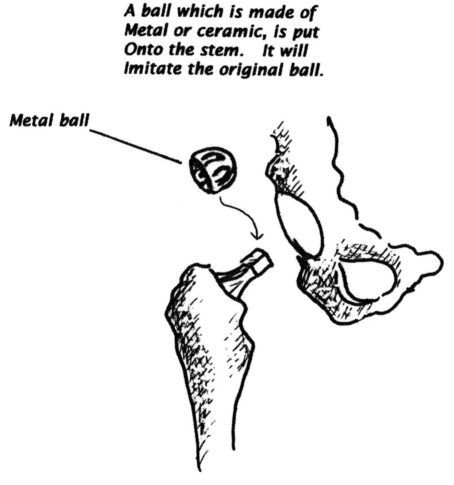

Figure 10.

The new ball and Socket are joined together

Figure 11.

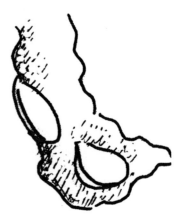

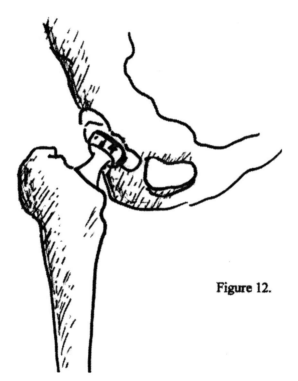

Figure 12.

Six

The Main Causes of Hip Problems

In the book called "Heal Your Hips," there are six main causes of hip problems described and listed. I found this information to be very valuable and it helped me to understand my own problem even more.

Osteoarthritis, the most common cause, was named as my problem by the hip replacement specialist. Osteoarthritis, the wearing down of the joints, affects millions of people worldwide. Some of the first signs of osteoarthritis in the hip could show up in the knee. One common problem often mentioned by people with this was not being able to lift one's leg into the car. Weakness and stiffness when walking or moving was a commonly described symptom.

Post traumatic arthritis, another cause, is very similar to Osteoarthritis. It occurs from injuries. Injury to an ankle or a knee could lead to a difference in leg length, which could end up causing arthritis in the hip because of the change in the normal way of walking. Injury to the lower back could even cause eventual hip damage. A fractured leg or ankle years before could alter one's gait and create eventual arthritis in the hip.

Rheumatoid arthritis inflicts devastating damage to the joints. It is an autoimmune disease in which the immune system attacks the tissues in the body.

Hip Dysplasia, which a person is born with, is usually diagnosed early in life, but not always. The mechanical function due to malformation in the hip joint causes the deteriorating problem.

Avascular Necrosis is the death of the bone due to the blood supply becoming unavailable to that joint. A common cause is trauma. Accidents that cause damage to the femoral head or dislocate the hip could cause damage to the blood vessels and result in bone death.

There are steroids, such as prednisone and cortisone, that can cause this problem. A physician prescribing these drugs to any patient should inform them of the risks. Alcoholism was also mentioned as a possible cause. When blood supply is cut off to the hip joint, the pain comes on abruptly. Pain in the groin and the front of the thigh can be intense. It also can seem to go away, but it may only be getting worse. The need to see a physician is important.

Soft-Tissue Injuries can include Tendonitis, Bursitis, Muscle strains, Capsulitis, Ligament Strains, and Muscle and Capsule contractures. All of these can affect one's hips. It would be wise to have a physician diagnose the problem to begin proper treatment.

Seven

The Compassion of the Hipsters

In contrast to the posts about surgical risks and problems, there was a great deal of hope and joy expressed at the Totally Hip Support Group: uplifting descriptions of joyous reconnections with life, new found abilities, and fulfillment in loved activities. There was humor. There were some jokes. There were intelligent questions asked, to which answers would often come from more than one source, so that you could compare possibilities. Encouragement and congratulations to fellow participants were also frequent. Empathy and compassion for those going through hard times was also a part of the daily climate at the Totally Hip Support Group. In my heart-felt quest to retain some of the things in my life that I felt were important to me, I began to ask human questions, rather than medical. With recognized vulnerability, my inquiries were stated. Everything I expressed was heard. Even things I did not mention about fear and change were addressed, as many of these people already knew what I was feeling before I could state it. They had walked the walk. They could answer questions before I ever asked. I continued to read the posts and dined with interest on everything I could get. My queries always received a response from more than one person. Some of the questions that I asked seemed petty to me, yet they were treated as though they were very substantial.

When directing a question to some of the women on the discussion Board about camping and how would they pee in the woods, two marvelous women shared with me their joys of camping. They loved their new hips and their new life. There was no joking around with how they described methods of urinating in the trees. One idea was leaning on a tree. Another was to keep a container handy, to urinate in while standing. A man on the discussion Board heard of an item on the market that women could use and stand while relieving themselves. Bashfulness did not seem to be a part of answering human questions.

The discussions were varied and ranged from having sex after surgery to the simple task of clipping your toenails after your Total Hip Replacement. Every bit of foresight that I could collect was welcomed. After reading posts from a kayacker, I personally sent a question about the knee to chest rule effecting how he enters his kayak. He informed me that his type of boat allows him to enter with ease, without having to bring his knee to his chest. The opening into his kayak was much larger than mine, which seemed to allow more ease for a hipster to embark.

There were some impressive accomplishments by hipsters that were discussed on the discussion Board. One woman had her black sash in martial arts four years after having a bilateral THR (bilateral means both hips). There were hipsters who were runners and swimmers, amongst others, who had a zest for the athletic aspects of life post-op. Many of the posts of such successes seemed to trigger hope that I, too, would remain active if I were to concede to this surgery.

The compassion shown on this discussion Board decreed that all of our feelings and concerns mattered. To learn what changes one could expect to make and to prepare to do whatever necessary to make these changes, both physically and emotionally, was priceless. The gift of being given a window to look into the personal lives of others who had taken on this surgical procedure was the best way I found to gain real insight.

My gratitude for the Hipsters increased with every experience I had with them. There was a longing in my heart to meet them. Their willingness to share information was far more valuable than what any doctor could tell me. The zest and gratitude for life and the reassurance that they projected into my consciousness convinced me that adversity in life can create tremendous growth, and perhaps too, I was growing in such ways. Many of them assured me that they were thrilled with their Total Hip Replacements and that they only had to change how they did certain things in order to be living a richer and more quality-filled life. Some of the posts about victories made me cry. Some of the posts about failure made me shudder. There was a truly human connection on this discussion Board. Warm comforts laced in fears prevailed in my understanding that I was not alone in this adventure. If I were to go for a bilateral THR, I would always have my family of hipsters. Someone would always be supportive and understanding as we would all be facing the positive gains, consequences, fears, and revisions from the THR.

Diagrams of The Total Hip Replacement Revision Surgery

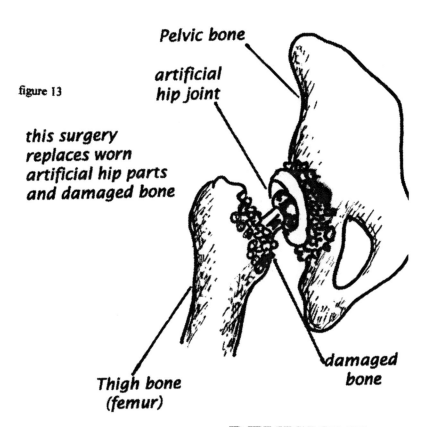

figure 13

Pelvic bone

artificial hip joint

this surgery replaces worn artificial hip parts and damaged bone

Thigh bone (femur)

damaged bone

With a Total Hip Replacement REVISIONS are Expected. The procedure is more complicated, as you Can see from the following drawings. Recovery time Is always longer and more difficult.

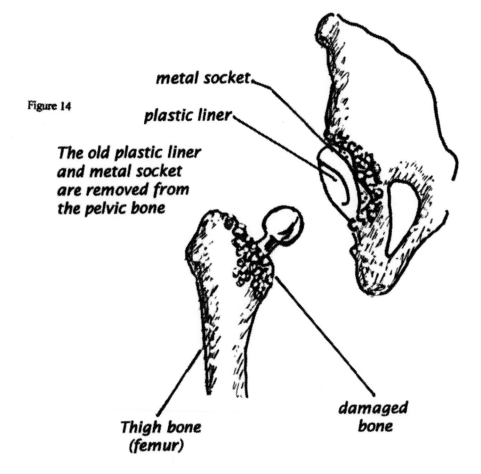

Figure 14

metal socket

plastic liner

The old plastic liner and metal socket are removed from the pelvic bone

Thigh bone (femur)

damaged bone

figure 15

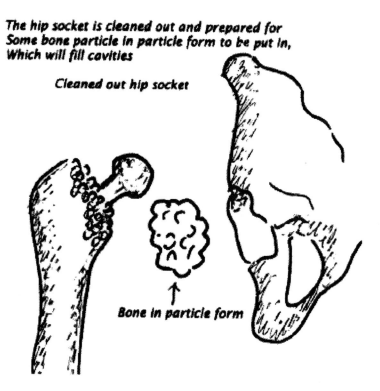

The hip socket is cleaned out and prepared for
Some bone particle in particle form to be put in,
Which will fill cavities

Cleaned out hip socket

Bone in particle form

figure 16

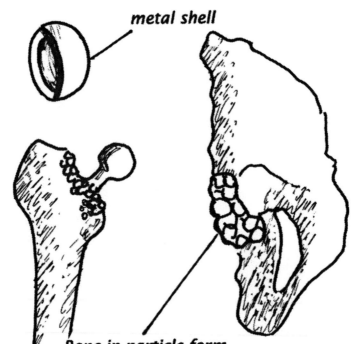

metal shell

Bone in particle form

figure 17

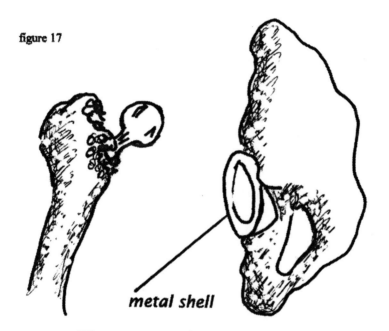

metal shell

The new metal socket is pressed into place. Screws may be used to secure the shell.

figure 18

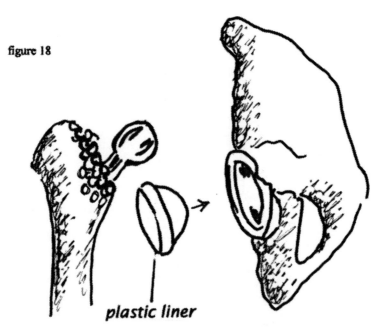

plastic liner

A new plastic, metal, or ceramic shell
Liner is pressed into place. Cement may be used.

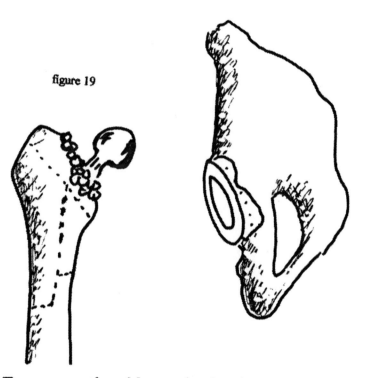

figure 19

To remove the old prosthesis, the
Bone around it may be cut into
Sections.   This is called an
"osteotomy".

figure 20

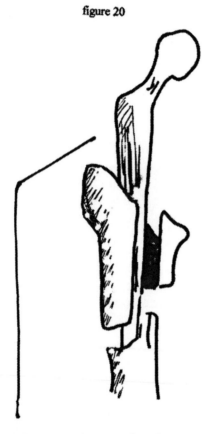
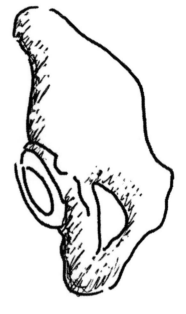

*Old metal prosthesis
being removed*

figure 21

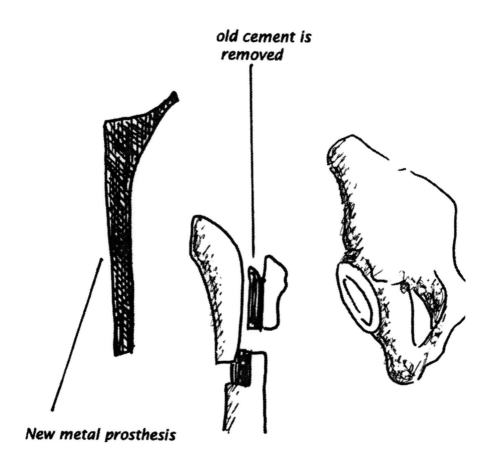

old cement is
removed

New metal prosthesis

figure 22

**New metal prosthesis is then pressed
or cemented into place**

**Wires hold the bone
together.**

new ball

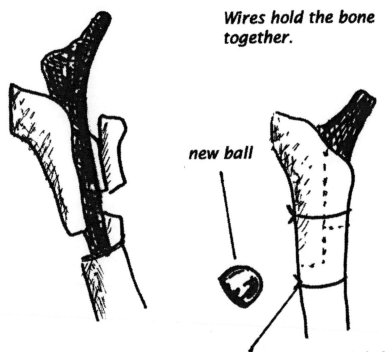

**Wire is used to close the segmented bone tightly
Around the metal component.   The wires may
Also help hold bone grafts in place for added
strength.**

figure 23

**A new metal or ceramic ball is placed on
The stem**

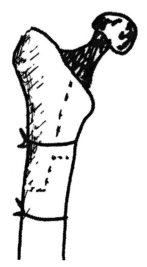

figure 24

**The ball and socket are joined together
To form a new hip joint**

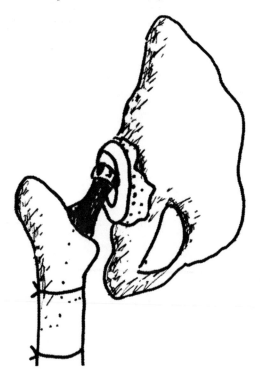

Eight

Searching For The Answer

Hoping to find a hip replacement surgeon who would be able to afford me more of what I wanted, I made an appointment with another doctor. I decided that I needed to go to someone who uses the larger ball that would reduce the chances of hip dislocation. Little did I know that I was about to discover something that would change my mind about seeing this doctor. I would later be canceling this appointment with a different avenue to travel to obtain what I needed for my life.

Meanwhile, I persuaded myself to search for someone who could replace cartilage. What a possibility! I knew that I needed to make some attempts to investigate all other possible avenues. This was to prevent regrets later, after taking on the irreversible Total Hip Replacement surgery.

Inquiries about hip donors and graftings were also made. I tried to leave no stone unturned. I read articles, ordered books, and searched the Internet.

One of the books that I mentioned earlier, "Heal Your Hips," was a valuable source of information. Within its pages, certain exercises were described that I could have done earlier in my life. These exercises could have possibly prevented the rapidness of the deterioration of my hips. In addition, nutritional care for the hips was discussed. In detail, a procedure called Hip Arthroscopy was described. I wanted to investigate Hip Arthroscopy after reading about it on the Totally Hip discussion Board.

The book described how the doctor employs a small scope and puts it through a tiny opening into the hip joint. Fragments in the joint, are removed. This type of treatment may help to prevent hip surgery in the future for some. The book enlightened me to the hereditary factors and how to recognize early signs of hip deterioration. I truly did not recognize my problems as symptoms of hip degeneration. I did not take into consideration that there had already been family members of mine who had to have hip replacements. In hindsight, this was possibly preventable.

Now, I faced the fact that there are no should haves or could haves. I was where I was, and had to keep putting one foot in front of the other in order to get my life back.

On the Totally Hip Discussion Board, a process called hip Resurfacing was mentioned. My first reaction to it was that I would not go the route of a guinea pig. It was considered to be experimental and investigational. My interest was triggered after reading some posts about its successes.

SECTION TWO

RESURFACING: THE BONE-SAVING TECHNIQUE

Nine
"Surfacehippies" Bringing Me Closer

It did not take long before I had read all about the Resurfacing process. Like the Hipsters having the Totallyhip Discussion Board, I found the Surfacehippy Discussion Board. By venturing into Surfacehippy@yahoogroups.com. It was here that I discovered a niche that brought me to some peace. Knowing that I could always go back to the hipsters, I felt that the Surfacehippies were more able to take me to the next step. Even though my love and respect would always remain with the Hipsters, my loyalties had to remain with my best interests: preserving everything I could that pertained to my health. In this case, my best interest was preserving the bone. Avoiding the total amputation of the head of the femur sounded attractive to me.

I eased my way into the Surface Hippy Discussion Board, where I became one of them. There seemed to be two groups on this Board: the more experienced searchers and the less experienced. Those who had the surgery were called the "Surfacehippies," and sometimes "Surfers." All seemed to be searching for answers and more information. Many were average people who became as scientists in researching the possibilities, outcomes, and probabilities of the Hip Resurfacing procedure.

I noted by observing the posts that an average person can become a scientist by facing the dark shadows created by pain and fear. The knowledge shared on this site was ever so valuable to my eventual decision. When humans bravely go where most doctors do not recommend is not a sign of ludicrousness and insanity. It is not a sign of rebellion. I saw it as a true statement of wanting the most life can offer and the willingness to become one of the trailblazers. The sustaining relationship that was easy for me to establish with the generous souls at the Surface Hippy Discussion Board was paramount. A person expressing their fear or a problem would receive many supportive responses. Some of the targets of discussion were physical pain, emotional pain, being simply terrified, clangy hip sounds, airport experiences, sexual activity after surgery, what's, when's, do's and don'ts, as well as surgery details such as number of stitches or where the cut was. Details on how to help choose a doctor were brought into perspective by the many posts.

We also discussed revisions for the Resurfacings. The topic of revisions was a serious subject. Revisions are do-overs. The Resurfacing procedure, as it is being done now, has been done in this way for eleven years in Europe, with an excellent track record. The logic, we determined, was that if an average Total Hip Replacement has to be revised every ten to fifteen years, then the track record of the Resurfacing technique is doing pretty well. One person on the Surfacehippy Discussion Board stated that if worse came to worse, we would have to get a Total Hip Replacement later, but just bought ourselves time to have a more active life. Buying time sounded like a good idea to me. According to some of the information gathered by the Surfacehippies, there is no reason for this to not last for twenty or thirty years, although guarantees are not possible.

Learning about the types of incisions that Surfacehippies receive from surgery further convinced me about the choice of my doctor. I learned from the Surfacehippy discussion Board that different doctors have different ways of making their incisions. Choosing a doctor who uses the posterolateral approach, which is from behind, would be important, as healing and physical therapy would go much more smoothly.
Sizes of incisions varied, according to the posts on the Board. The smallest that I was made aware of was five and three quarter inches. It seemed that many were longer, perhaps an average of twelve inches.

There were some people on the Board who were concerned about scars and how they would look in a bathing suit. Discussions about which creams and oils would be best to eliminate the obviousness of the scar brought forth ideas on looking better, but I did not care. I wanted to look fit, but a scar, or two scars in my case, would be representative of a pain free life and would be welcomed.

"Surfing" for information (as the Surfacehippies describe it) about the three devices used for this procedure was my next endeavor. The three that I found were all metal on metal: the BHR (Birmingham Hip Replacement), Cormet 2000, and the Conserve Plus. All three sounded effective and it seemed to be a matter of where you live, or where you go for the surgery, as to which device you would get. In the USA, you would get a Conserve or Cormet, while in other parts of the world you would get the BHR or Cormet. They are not identical. If you are large boned or have complications and have surgery in the USA, then you could possibly end up with a Total Hip Replacement at this point in time (Jan, 2003), because the FDA has not completed the trials and there is not a full range of parts available yet in the US. But, that will change when the trials are completed.

As they say, "the proof is in the pudding." When comparing the stories of Surfacehippies, all three of the types of devices that I read about seemed to be beneficial. I did not feel qualified to make a choice in the debates on which device was superior. Instead, I felt more confident that if I chose a doctor who was successful in this field, I would be making the right choice overall with whatever device he used. It seemed to me that once you have weighed all of the factors that are important to you in choosing your doctor, you have to invest trust into your relationship with this person. Knowing that their abilities are a continuance of experiential knowledge, you will have to rely on their choice of which device to use and how to use it. The first key though, I felt, was a careful evaluation. The Surfacehippies helped this to be possible.

Ten

FDA Study/Risks

A subject that frequented the Discussion Board was the subject of insurance companies. Because the procedure is not FDA approved in the United States, insurance companies did not always cover the surgery. Many people were in the stages of appealing, some being approved, and others just giving up to either having a THR or paying out of pocket for the Resurfacing procedure. "Experimental" and "investigational" were the two words used by insurance companies due to the incomplete FDA study. A simple phone call to my insurance company verified that I was most likely going to be denied unless my appeal was effective.

I became aware of another concern, which was the metal ions in the blood caused from a metal on metal implant. One of the questions that some of the Surfacehippy posts reflected was about the cancer risk caused by the metal ions. It seemed that even though the hardness of the metal would not be expected to wear like other materials that are used for hips implants, the question still existed of what effect the metal would have on the body. Perhaps the upcoming results of the FDA trials would reveal this information. It was noted that many studies were being conducted, and many people have all ready had such metal in their bodies for a number of years without known problems.

The two metals that sparked concern were cobalt and chromium.
Cobalt is a necessary element for the body and can be found in the liver and kidneys. It is also in foods items. If there is an excess of cobalt in the system, the kidneys' function is to eliminate it. Chromium also is essential to the body. A deficiency of it can create high glucose levels. The effects of high levels of Chromium in the body were not established, thus, the studies.

It was suggested to use anti-oxidant formulas or Vitamin C, which is an anti-oxidant, to help eliminate some of the metal ions from the body. On the Surfacehippy discussion Board, someone mentioned that one could donate a unit of blood every eight weeks to dilute the metal ions flowing through the body. Another idea was to have the kidney functions checked before surgery. I never found any information about people having kidney functions checked.

One obvious idea if you were concerned about metal ions would be to have your drinking water tested to see if it is high in such metals, and use bottled water if it is. It would be sensible to also check your multi-vitamins/minerals to make sure that you are not taking any cobalt or chromium.

With the task of weighing the risks, it was my privilege to decide which route was better. I had the choice of taking pain-killers and remaining in a deteriorating state until I could get my insurance company to assist in paying for the surgery. The pain-killers would be possibly harmful to my bone quality, as well as my kidneys and liver, and waiting was seriously jeopardizing my spine. The second choice was to go for the Total Hip Replacement, which I had already ruled out. The third choice was to have the Hip Resurfacing surgery in a timely fashion and be able to not only walk again and regain my normal activities, but to also be able to maintain spinal health. It was a medical necessity.

Like many of the other Surfacehippies, I tried to find out how close the FDA was to approving this procedure. Perhaps approval was right around the corner. When reading the posts on the Board about the experiences of others and their attempts to find out, I learned that the information we wanted was not easy to acquire. One of the representatives of Wright Technologies, the maker of the Conserve Plus resurface device and responsible for the clinical trials, stated that the FDA trial is probably in its final phase and then it could take as many as two years for final FDA approval. Meanwhile, the studies are going on. I read some postings that referred to these studies and the need for successes. Thus, it seemed to some of the Surfacehippies that some of the surgeons in this country may be more conservative than others in their choice of patients. It is possible that the doctors would only want patients those who could guarantee good results by not having a complicated hip problem. This situation created a fear among those of us with a more complicated hip problem of waking up with a Total Hip Replacement if our cases were difficult.

After reading about some U.S. doctors who did not speak of increased activity levels that one would have with a resurface device as opposed to a Total Hip Replacement, I began to compare stories. There were stories of Surfacehippies who have returned to martial arts, water skiing, snow skiing, bungee jumping, judo, tennis, yoga, Pilates, rock climbing, and so on. I felt sad to realize the possibility that a doctor would not tell someone about the wonderful capabilities that the Hip Resurfacing procedure could bring. Courtrooms and lawsuits have induced fears which limit our doctors in many ways. With the eventual FDA approval, I knew that this would change.

Diagrams Of The Hip Resurfacing Procedure

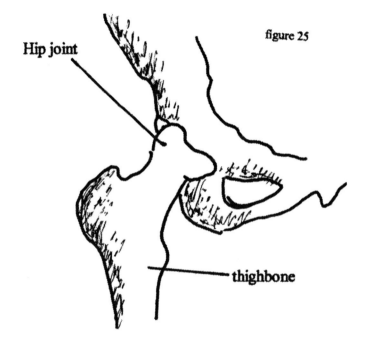

Hip joint

figure 25

thighbone

swarminteractive.com/orthopedic/interactive

figure 26

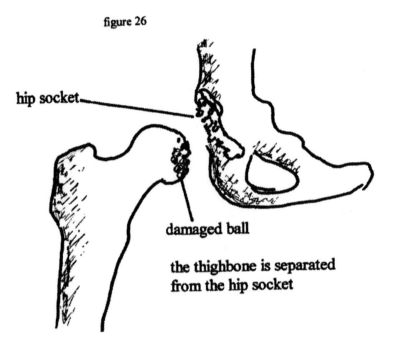

hip socket

damaged ball

the thighbone is separated
from the hip socket

**strong bone in
the femoral head
is necessary to
support the
resurfacing
device**

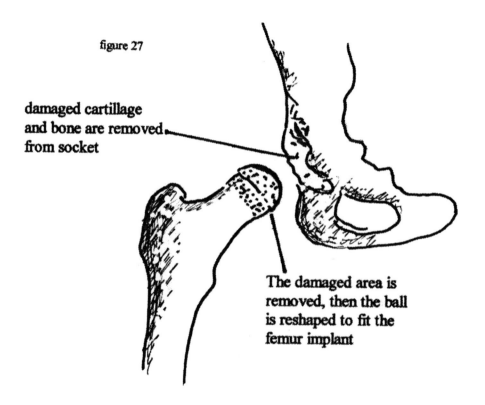

figure 27

damaged cartillage
and bone are removed
from socket

The damaged area is
removed, then the ball
is reshaped to fit the
femur implant

The femoral head is preserved.

figure 28

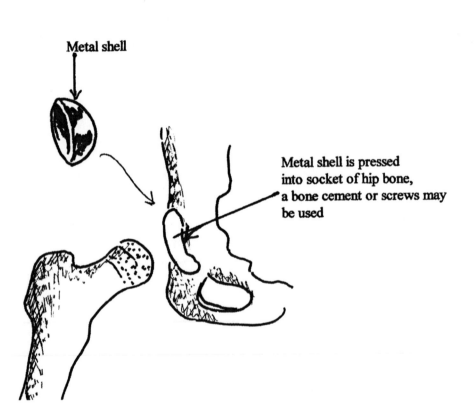

Metal shell

Metal shell is pressed
into socket of hip bone,
a bone cement or screws may
be used

figure 29

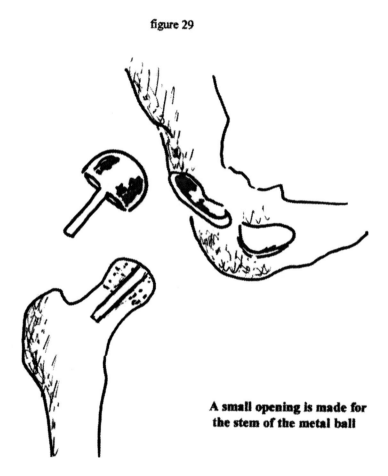

**A small opening is made for
the stem of the metal ball**

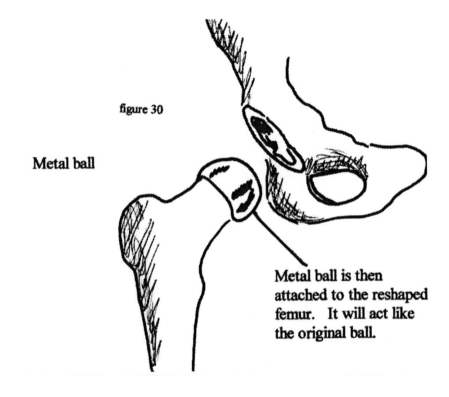

figure 30

Metal ball

Metal ball is then attached to the reshaped femur. It will act like the original ball.

Figure 31

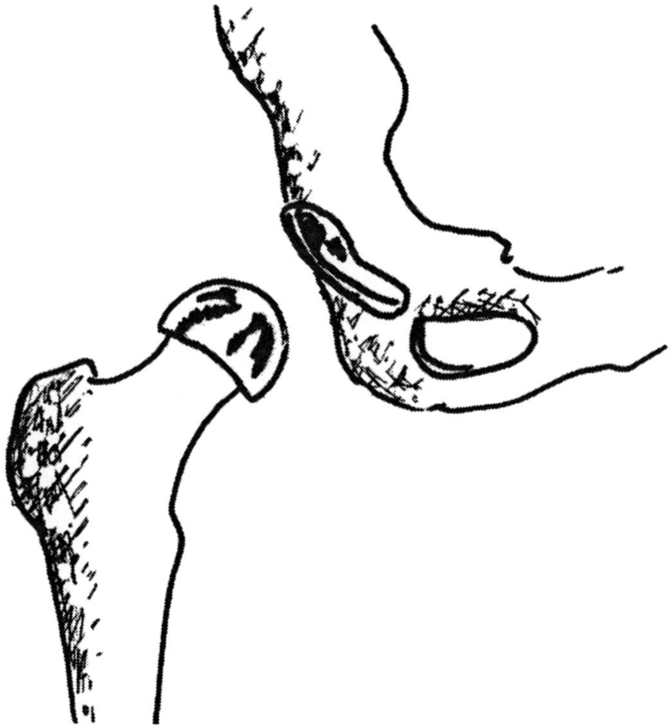

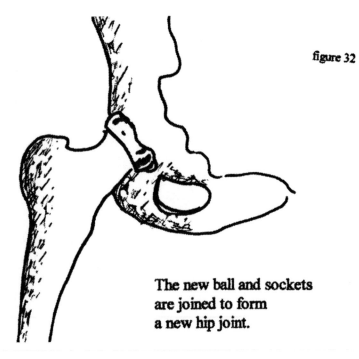

figure 32

The new ball and sockets
are joined to form
a new hip joint.

Eleven

The Not So Hip Set Back

My choice of doctors was influenced by the Surfacehippies. My X-rays were sent to him and we had a telephone interview. It all seemed so simple. He submitted paperwork to my insurance company.

Within a few weeks, the first denial letter from my insurance company arrived. They recommended that I receive a Total Hip Replacement. The very thought of the limitations that a Total Hip Replacement would afford me made the entire situation seem insane. Their reason for the denial of coverage for the Resurfacing was because it was investigational and experimental. I had read on the Board of other Surfacehippies who had been approved by their insurance carriers. Surely persistence would be the answer, and to not take "no" for an answer! It was now time for the first appeal. I had to make my first appeal with little assistance from my doctor, and really did not know how to do it. My doctor sent a letter to me to include with my appeal.

By asking for help from the Surfacehippies on the Board, I was endowed with numerous possibilities that could be used to prepare the paperwork. Some of them mailed me samples that I could model my own appeal after. One of them proofread for me. Through their guidance, I prepared my first appeal. It included information on how the Resurfacing would eliminate any further damage to the spine. It included letters from two doctors explaining the condition of the spine and the way the hips were creating more problems. It explained how my income came from teaching Pilates. The appeal showed how I would be able to continue with this career with a Resurfacing procedure. The appeal also detailed how the Resurfacing would most likely prevent the multiple spinal fusions that were predicted for me, as well as the cost of pain management.

Longevity was also an issue. Many of my family members maintained their health into a ripe old age. This fact alone could contribute to the problem of forcing me to have many revisions over the years and ending up in a wheelchair during the last part of my life. The common knowledge of dislocation possibilities with a Total Hip Replacement was also made into an issue. The letter from my doctor mentioned how my active life would greatly benefit from the Resurfacing procedure and would be hindered by a Total Hip Replacement. When I felt satisfied that the appeal was complete, I sent it in. Within two weeks, I received a letter from my insurance carrier. Tension surrounded me as I fumbled to open the envelope. It came to me like a dark messenger. The letter was one of denial and concluded that I was eligible for a Total Hip Replacement through their insurance coverage. The Resurface procedure was described to be investigational and experimental.

Of course, I had a lot of nerve to think that I could do the appeal process simply, when many others had to appeal numerous times and struggle with the process. At that time, in my estimation, one of the best tips given to me by the discussion Board was to find a surgeon who employs people to deal with the insurance providers. They "speak" insurance. They know the methods that work.

One of the people on the Board said that insurance companies make more money when they say "no" at first. It seemed that persistence in appealing had proven to bring about good results. Thus, I decided that the doctor I had first chosen was not the best doctor for my situation. His staff did not seem to be heavily involved in making the appeals happen.

On the discussion Board, I had been reading about another doctor in Maryland. There were many posts about how his insurance person had been very successful in getting approvals from the insurance carriers for the Resurfacing surgery. It would not cost me anything to have my records transferred to his office. With a simple phone call, I had all of my records sent and the insurance wizard began working on my appeal. To help assure a better chance of success, I sent paperwork that included how my Pilates teaching career needed to be considered, as a Total Hip Replacement would end it. I sent photos of me teaching the class along with letters pertaining to this situation from my doctor, my chiropractor, and the gym where I taught Pilates. I was told that my appeal was hopeful.

This appeal took a lot longer than the first one. Anxieties did not allow much rest for me, and I emailed the doctor's office frequently to see if they had heard anything. Patience was always recommended to me. More than three months had passed. A time measured in how I could stay out of pain and continue my life. Finally the letter of denial came like an ogre out of the darkest grotto, to gloat that I would not be able to have my life back. In this letter, they again recommended that I receive the Total Hip Replacement. The bone saving Resurfacing procedure was denied.

With the knowledge that I would only be allowed to make three appeals, I knew that the last appeal to my insurance company had to be effective.

With the encouragement that I received from the Surfacehippy Board, I decided to go ahead with my third appeal with great care and creativity. I asked for more advise on the Board. It was not long before I received an envelope of paperwork from two of the Surfacehippies who had appealed to their insurance company and had put a lot of information together. The time consuming process of assembling the third appeal was influenced by my burning desire to regain my life. Included in this booklet was detailed and complete information about the Resurfacing procedure. Showing how this surgery would save the insurance company money by eliminating the possible spinal fusions was also a consideration. The diligent work that I put into the appeal was laced with prayers and hopes. I included pages of exercises (with photos) from a Pilates book showing that a very high percentage of the exercises I needed to do consisted of the knee coming near the chest, which would be breaking the ninety degree rule, which could cause a dislocation of the Total Hip Replacement prosthesis. I felt that someone on the appeals Board would see the possibility of career-hindering limitations that the amputations of the balls of my hips could create.

The insurance company responded quickly to my appeal. Within two weeks, a letter of denial was sent to me. Their letter stated: "The appeals process has been exhausted, therefore additional information will not be considered for review." What it meant to me was that I was truly on my own.

Some of the people on the Board encouraged me to appeal again. There was one man who made eight appeals before he was finally approved. Another man went personally to the appeals board meeting of his insurance company to make his appeal in person. He was approved. There were possibilities involving persistence, but I could not go on in my deteriorating condition.

At this point, it was medically necessary for me to act. Depression was present everyday, as my life was limited to a reclining chair. Walking was the enemy to my spine. When I did walk, it was only when necessary and it caused further trauma to the back problem. I could no longer sleep in bed. My muscles were atrophying. I was becoming weaker. The challenges of finding ways to alleviate pain were futile.

Twelve

The Option to Fly to Europe

Many Americans were traveling abroad to have the Hip Resurfacing Procedure. Numerous stories on the Board made it clear to me that one of the major reasons was due to the insurance company denials for coverage. When having to pay out of pocket, people were finding it to be much more attractive to pay the lower prices of European surgeries and to also have wonderful doctors. The cost in Belgium, for instance, was approximately one third of the cost in the United States. In England, the cost was also markedly lower. The Surfacehippies on the discussion Board were not shy about telling how much they paid.

Another reason that certain Americans choose to go to Europe was because they were told by their doctor in America that they were not eligible for the Resurfacing surgery. The surgeons in Belgium and England were discussed frequently, and I was drawn to Dr. Koen De Smet in Belgium because he had the reputation of taking on the tough cases with success. I wanted to have two hips done simultaneously. the choice was simple. Success stories of the European surgeries were numerous.

On some of the posts discussions were about the pros and cons of having this surgery done in the United States in comparison to Europe. It seemed that a number of the patients in the United States were kept on crutches much longer than the European Resurfacing patients. This seemed to me to go hand in hand with the fear of liability in our American setting, or the extra care taken to assure the success of the study.

The posts about the surgeon in Belgium impressed me deeply. Reading about him on his website convinced me further. His use of the posterior approach in surgery, which eliminates the cutting of muscles, was preferred. I emailed Dr. De Smet in Belgium. He answered within a day and I was sending my X-rays by overnight mail. There was also the consideration that I could have both hips done at the same time. Being in constant contact with two of his patients who had both hips resurfaced simultaneously, was a guidepost for my decision.

Upon receiving my X-rays, Dr. De Smet informed me by email that I was indeed a candidate for the Resurfacing technique. He also agreed to work his magic on both of my hips at the same time. Remembering someone on the Board getting their appointment for surgery scheduled in a two-week period, I mentioned that I could be in Ghent, at the hospital, in two weeks. He informed me that he was going on a vacation and told me that my surgery could not happen for six weeks. Sigh. He also mentioned that he did not want me to take any anti-inflammatories. The date he gave me for surgery was September 11, 2002. I asked him for a different date. My reasoning was due to the significance of that date to many. He responded that I would be fine in Belgium on that date. I was putty in his hands.

I was blessed that I could borrow the money, as many others were forced to do. I felt sad for those who could not get their hands on the funds. The number of Americans flying to foreign shores to have this gift of choice was amazing to me. It was thrilling to become a part of this group, braving an operation that was not recommended by most physicians in their homeland, but was honored by much of the world.

On the Surfacehippy discussion Board, I discovered that I already had a roommate for my hospital stay. She was from the west coast and was having one hip done. We chatted on the site and learned a little about each other. There were also some others who were going to Belgium at the same time, with surgery dates within ten days of my own. Our little discussions in America gave me plans to meet these people in person while over there. It was exciting to think that I would actually be able to connect each of them with a face.

The fact was that I would be only the fourth patient of Dr. De Smet to have the Bilateral Hip Resurfacing (two hips in the same surgery).

With the grace of the Discussion Board, the two Bilateral Surfacehippies that I connected with helped me a great deal. One of the two was a woman, who pretty much had to depend on herself. She did it alone. Why couldn't I? She became my double hip sis. Her advise to me was to try to get someone to accompany me. She helped me to assess all of the pros and cons, and it definitely weighed out in favor of having a helper. The other person was a man, who also had both hips done simultaneously. His experiences convinced me that I would be pretty much disabled if I had both of them done at the same time. Through the generosity of these two, I had an idea of what to expect. What I had chosen to endure was to be far more difficult than the one hippers, as I would soon see. They helped me to prepare myself mentally for this difficult procedure by fueling my knowledge of what to expect.

When I posed the question onto the Discussion Board about going alone, many voices came forth (in writing, of course) saying that it would be so much better to have a helper. They assured me that I would need an extensive amount of assistance. The reasons they gave were sound and I accepted the offer of my closest friend and sweetheart, D'Jango, who wanted to come with me.

Thirteen

The Whats and Whys of Preparations

From reading the posts on the Board daily, I realized that I was not doing everything that I could to prepare myself for surgery. Eliminating pain medications to maintain bone quality was not enough. Taking vitamins and calcium was not enough either. My crime was allowing myself to fall into such an inactive state that my body had become weakened. Strong arms would be needed to get in and out of bed after surgery. Upper body strength would be needed to handle crutches. Maintaining some mobility in my body would help me to heal faster. My decision to begin swimming every morning at a friend's pool was a good one. Every morning, with a cautious and slow pace, I would immerse myself into the experience of water exercise. Indulging in every exercise that did not afflict me with unbearable pain, I noticed within a very short time that my strength and mobility were improving. My mental and emotional states were also better.

Preparations meant remaining in contact with the Surfacehippy Board everyday. A surgery in Belgium would require more preparations than one in my own country. The experiences of the Surfacehippies who had gone to Belgium for their surgery (often called the Belgium Hippies) brought me information on how to get the hotel prices lowered. Being educated about finding the best plane fares, where and what to eat in Belgium, places to stay, how to take the train to Ghent, how to convert money to Eurodollars, how to check into the hospital, as well as tidbits about raised toilet seats relieved a lot of pressure from my weary mind. My hospital stay was to be three days longer than most of the one hippers. Descriptions from the "Belgium Hippies" of the not so wonderful hospital food were accompanied with the remedies of where to have your special someone get you food. I prepared a notebook of information.

Well before my departure for surgery, I obtained a handicap placard to hang in my car to use during recovery. Preparing to be disabled was a creative venture. A raised toilet seat was recommended. Elbow crutches were also a suggestion. Buying a reacher to pick things up with during the early weeks after surgery, putting a non-slippery bath mat in the shower, and having items in the kitchen and bathroom put into an easy to reach place was a part of considering what life would be like on crutches. Another plan was to use a backpack to carry things from one place to another as my crutch-busy hands would be unavailable for carrying things. I put a bar stool in the kitchen so I could put fruits and vegetables on it and slide it across with my crutches to transport produce to the cutting Board.

Cutting toenails before surgery was a must, as I realized I would not be touching my toes for several weeks. Fingernail polish would be removed before surgery, so I did not bother putting any on.

I truly had become one with this group of beings without faces calling themselves the "Belgium Hippies." The Belgium Hippies were not the only ones who gave me wonderful information for my preparations. The American Hippies, the England Hippies, and Hippies from other parts of the world were all an aid to me, through the grace of the Discussion Board. Without them, I would have most likely lost out on the best that was available to me.

Knowing that I had to be completely prepared for the experience, and visualizing the different possibilities that I would encounter, many questions manifested. Answers and ideas were returned. Ordering wheelchair assistance with the plane tickets was of great importance. There were the obvious questions and then there were the more personal questions. It was so fitting that the only other female Belgium Hippy who had both hips resurfaced at the same time made herself available for my queries. In trying to imagine how I would use the toilet on the long plane trip back to America, maneuvering with two crutches, unable to bend or sit on anything low, her solution was inventive and simple. For a woman, she advised, it would be easier to not wear underwear and to wear a long loose skirt. The absence of shyness when it came to important details was helpful.

The valuable advise of upgrading my ticket to business class seat for the trip home made coping much easier. The ability to lay back in the business class seat and having a foot rest was also a suggestion of my doctor, who stated that for me to sit upright for long periods of time would increase possibilities of swelling.

I ordered a book on how to prepare for surgery. The book offered ideas for emotional, physical, and spiritual preparations. From it, I learned how to prepare a tape of healing and positive thoughts. Using my voice to create a thirty-minute cassette abundant with positive thoughts and uplifting background music did not take much time. It was worthwhile for the moments that I was going to be writhing and impatient. I also acquired a cassette of calming classical music.

My passport was ready. My tickets were in order. My payment to the doctor was completed.

Overseas Surfacehippies are told that phone cards can be purchased over there. Remembering address books and email addresses was also important. Packing my own soap and toothpaste, as well as normal cosmetics and other toiletries was common sense. I did not realize that later I would wish for a bit of laundry soap to wash out my compression stockings.

Crutches were an item that some hippies thought important to plan ahead for. In the United States, elbow crutches cost eighty-seven dollars, while in Europe they were seventeen dollars. The decision to get crutches in Europe was a simple one, as my doctor suggested getting them there.

One woman on the Surfacehippy site wore a special air filter around her neck to help with the cigarette smoke in Europe. I did not worry about that.

Due to the priceless foreknowledge of what was in store for me, I realized that loose clothing was going to be my best style. Baggy dresses that I could pull over my head and would not require me to bend, loose skirts, baggy shorts or pants (drawstrings) two sizes too large would be best. I was told to avoid elastic waistbands, since they can create discomfort when pulling them on as they tend to push the knees together. Knowing that I would be fine using the hospital gowns, I did not pack a lot of nightgowns. Using hospital gowns would eliminate having to worry about laundry.

A pair of good walking shoes was highly recommended. Remembering that I would be taking my first steps in these shoes, and that I needed to be safe, I decided to leave my flip-flops at home. I took some sturdy, comfortable shoes that would be easy to slip on and off. Checking my shoes for skid proof soles was also a good suggestion by the Surfacehippies. I knew that I would not need many socks because I would be wearing two compression stockings.

When I inquired about the subject of taking underwear, one woman stated that she used thongs so that the underpants did not interfere with her incisions. Several did not use underwear. If you consider that you may be swollen, you may not be able to use your underpants.

There were so many suggestions about what to take and I noted the ones that I felt to be most important. Insurance papers and papers for admission were items of importance to remember. I did pack my own special neck pillow. One woman mentioned that she took her spongy mattress pad. Other suggestions were a cheap watch or alarm clock, normal cosmetics and mirror, headache medication (as many of the Surfacehippies experienced headaches right after surgery), gentle laxative, medications that you need to be taking (making sure your doctor knows about these), a good book, and a journal and pen.

I was told not to take expensive or irreplaceable jewelry. Watches fell into that category. These items could be misplaced or even stolen in the hospital.

One suggestion startled me in the "Heal Your Hips" book. It was to use a black felt pen to write "NO" on the good hip and "THIS HIP" on the one to have surgery. Just the concept of a surgeon operating on the wrong hip is a disturbing one, but the truth is that foresight is better than hindsight. Of course, in my situation with two hips going under the knife, I did not have to worry about that.

I also packed a large plastic garbage bag, as some of the other Hippies used one to sit on and slide into an automobile without dragging their stitches. I was told to make sure it is carefully removed after you are situated for safety sake. This idea came in handy for many in the hospital also, as when trying to move incisions across the sheets to get out of bed, one would appreciate ways to avoid pain.

Often, blood is taken in advance to store for the day of surgery in case you need it. I was prepared to begin this process, as did other American Hippies. I was informed by my doctor that I did not need to worry about that.

Fourteen

The Long Flight To The Operating Room

We flew out of Corpus Christi and into Dallas, where we would be making our connection to Brussels. In Dallas, our time was limited. We needed to get to our gate. We could not find a courtesy cart to help us in our haste. Regardless of my inability to walk fast, I began to limp quickly toward our destination. D'Jango grabbed one of the luggage carts, which are similar in appearance to a grocery store shopping cart without the top basket. He had me sit on the base, near the floor, holding our carry-ons. He ran through the airport pushing me. We traveled fast. My hair was blowing. It was funny to see how people reacted as we breezed by. We arrived at the point where we could get the tram to our gate quickly.

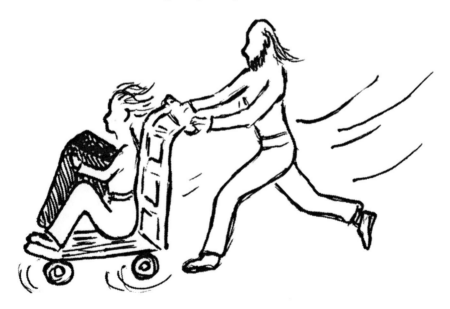

Figure 32

The flight to Brussels went well. The wheelchair assistance was wonderful and got us through all of the lines without problems. Packing lightly made it much easier.

Upon our arrival in Brussels, I merely had to follow the directions given to me on the Surfacehippy Board to know where to go next. Taking in the wonderful sights of this beautiful Belgium city was a delight, even though each step was a reminder of the real reason I was there.

We traveled to Ghent, which was where the hospital was located. The old city of Ghent, which is built on canals and bathed in history, seemed to welcome us. The people were friendly and offered directions when we needed them. After arriving at the hospital, I stood outside feeling vulnerable and afraid. Here I was, a woman who originally thought she could do this alone, wanting to run away, yet, could hardly walk. D'Jango helped me with encouraging words. Together, we walked into the hospital where I was checked in.

The hospital appeared to be well seasoned. The obvious unimportant things, such as walls that were somewhat battered, floors that had seen years of use, and hospital furnishings that were obviously used for a long time, were not vital. What counted was that I was in good hands. The staff spoke English and the care was excellent. I went to my room, and noticed that each of the two beds had extra pillows for my roommate and I. People with hip problems often figure out that sleeping with a pillow between knees can make all the difference. It was nice to feel that they were going to accommodate our needs. My roommate had not arrived yet. The nurses chatted with me while taking blood work, my blood pressure, etc. They also took new X-rays.

Knowing that I was going to have my first meeting with Dr. Koen De Smet, I should have prepared a list of questions. When I met him face to face, I forgot many of the things that I wanted to ask. From that experience I would advise others to always have their queries written out. It did not matter at that point as I had all of my major concerns addressed by the doctor on the Internet well in advance.

We discussed the length of the surgery, the amount of time he felt I would be in the recovery room, but mostly, I wanted to just connect with him. I liked everything about him. Again, I was putty in his hands, and grateful for it.

We discussed anesthetic and he recommended that I receive both an epidermal as well as an anesthetic due to me having two hips done. This was indeed more than his patients having one hip done would get. They would only get the anesthetic, but then, of course, I would be in surgery at least twice the time and having the double whammy.

Expecting to see my hospital roommate and her family, as described to me by email on the Surfacehippy discussion Board, led me to such a group in the admitting room. We hugged and shared the moment of the beginning of our great adventure. We were both scheduled for surgery on the following morning. I watched her walk and noticed how her right hip was very unlevel.

In the evening we were give further preparations, and that included an enema. We were not to eat or drink after midnight. My roommate's husband brought us both a dessert. It felt like a strange sort of celebration, with bits of fear and concerns mixed with huge hopes and plans of regaining our lives. Falling asleep was difficult and we talked for a couple of hours.

The night seemed long. I could not sleep for many hours. I listened to my Walkman and used the tape of positive thoughts that I made for myself, as well as some classical music. The headphones made it possible for me to listen without disturbing my roommate. I kept the Walkman under my blanket to further honor the silence of the darkened room. I was very vigilant about not making noise when turning the cassette tape over to the other side. It was 6 am before I knew it. Did I sleep at all last night? It was only eleven p.m. in

Texas now, I thought. I wondered if my daughters, who lived in different parts of Texas, were still awake. Maybe not.

While my roommate and I waited, she told me of her experiences of climbing very tall mountains. It seemed to me that this was one of the tall mountains of her life to climb. We again shared our hopes and fears with each other.

As they rolled her bed out of the room for surgery, I wished her well, as she also wished me well, "Good luck!" I would be following after her. I was grateful that I did have an early morning surgery, as we were not supposed to drink any water before surgery. I was already very thirsty. I felt grateful that I was not one of the afternoon patients. If I would give anyone advise about this, I would tell them to request a morning surgery in the very beginning when the scheduling is done.

The nurses came for me at nine a.m. I spent one hour in the pre-op preparation room, where both of my legs were swabbed with disinfectant, shaved, and intravenous medications amongst other preparations were made. I enjoyed hearing the nurses speak to the other patients in different languages.

After about an hour, they wheeled me into the operating room. All I remember was that it was cold and everything seemed to be stainless steel, high tech, shiny, and clean. My life was about to change.

Fifteen

Three Hours and Two Devices Later

My surgery lasted for three hours, which, from what I learned on the Board, is typical in Belgium for a bilateral resurfacing. The single hip surgeries usually last for under an hour. My roommate's was forty-five minutes. Forty-five minutes to change her entire life! Three hours to change mine!

I slightly remember the recovery room. I thought it was too hot. They were caring for me and kept a warm bubble blanket over me. I remember saying that I was hot and a loving voice spoke to me saying that they needed to keep me warm. Being mostly unconscious during the three hour recovery room period, I was told that it was longer than most. One of the reasons was because I happened to lose a couple of units of blood. They gave me blood.

When they rolled me out of the recovery room, I was awake. D'Jango was waiting for me. I was coherent, but very sleepy.

Later that day, my doctor smiled as he came into my room to explain to me how the operation went. He mentioned that I was given two units of blood. He told me that my left hip, the one which was deteriorated to the greatest degree, was more difficult one to work on. He explained that I ended up getting two different sized hips. The one on the left was commonly a man's size, as the bone was thicker. He said that the prosthesis on the right side was commonly a woman's size, somewhat smaller. He said that I will never notice it. Some adults receive a child size if they are small, which I discovered later that my roommate received. He brought one of the BHR implants with him to show me. I held it. It probably weighed a pound. I marveled at the fact that two of these shiny charms were to change my life.

Regardless of how I felt, the physical therapist massaged my legs and moved them gently from the very beginning. He had me do some resistance exercises as he carefully secured my legs, one at a time.

For the first 24 hours, I was running a fever while my one hip sister was up and walking, 100% weight bearing, with the aid of a walker.

I was on a catheter and would remain so for two days. Despite what I remembered reading on the Board from other Surfacehippies who did not like being catheterized, I was glad to have it, as it relieved me of the worry of having to get up to pee or to have to use an uncomfortable bed pan. I had low blood pressure and had to keep my legs elevated. I remembered reading that many doctors catheterize their patients because the anesthetic causes your body to not realize when your bladder is full. I guess the uncatheterized One-Hippers did not have that problem as they were up and walking on the first day. Their mobility was astounding to me. They were going to the cafeteria in the hospital for lunch, socializing, and already enjoying their new hips. I remembered one man saying that he wished he would have saved time for sightseeing in Belgium after his surgery when he did not hurt so much. Instead he did his sightseeing pre-op and in pain.

The first few nights post-op were very difficult. I remembered the descriptions on the Board about the first two nights for the Two-Hippers. It was not easy for them, either. Fever, low blood pressure, dizziness, weakness, effects from the morphine drip, and helplessness brought to my mind how my double whammy Surfacehippy friends from the Board told me that they could not wait for the first few days to be over. The need to move to find comfort only brought frustration. Using the bedpan was a major episode and I needed help in all aspects.

The physical therapist was slow at getting me onto my feet due to my dizziness and weakened state. He assisted me with gentle exercises that I could do on my back. It was not until day three that I was up on my feet. That was the day that my roommate was preparing to leave the hospital and go to the hotel. She was walking quite well. It was at this time that I would begin to hear the stories of the One-Hippers going out to see the sights using only one crutch, while I remained confined.

Just to slide my body to the edge of the bed was difficult. I was so weak. When my buttocks were dragging on the sheets creating friction and irritating my incisions, I remembered the garbage bag. By slipping it under me, I could easily slide across the bed.

My first moment on my feet was frightening as I was weak and still a bit dizzy. But I did notice something different. It did not hurt when I stood. I was putting 100 % weight on both of my new hips. They walked me to a chair, which was only about five feet away. I sat in it on a soft pillow for about fifteen minutes. This experience was just the breaking of the ice for what was to come, for everyday I would be getting better.

Truly, I felt blessed that I did not have the nauseous or migraine headaches like some of the others described on the Board. By day five, I noticed a big change. I managed to get up by myself and take little walks without the physical therapist being present. I felt markedly better, even though the walks in the halls exhausted me. I suppose my anemic condition contributed to that. I still used a walker. My walker had become my trusty friend. It gave me a form of independence. It seemed abrupt when the therapist switched me to the elbow crutches.

The elbow crutches did not go under the armpits. Instead, you gripped a handle with your lower arm put through the top loop on the crutch, thus the name. I was a little wobbly at first learning to use them. The therapist said that elbow crutches were far better for me than the standard crutches.

While walking slowly in the hospital hall with my two crutches, I was delighted to visit the three other Americans that I already knew from the Surfacehippy discussion Board. They were there for surgery on the day before I left the hospital. It was so much fun meeting them face to face after sharing so many communications online. They were noticeably anxious about their upcoming surgery.

There was pain. Some of it kept me up at night. I really did not hear about anyone having terrible pain. My worst pain was from having to stay on my back and not being able to move about. My heels were getting sores from being in constant contact with the sheets. It may sound strange, but that was my major complaint in the pain department. I remember wishing I had some soft foam rubber pads to put under them. Even the softest pillow was not soft enough.

The physical therapist came daily to my hotel room, as he had when I was in the hospital. Every day he would massage my legs for about twenty minutes, then he would help me move my legs into bending and various positions. He taught me exercises that I was to do at home, since I would not have a physical therapist in America. Every day, the therapist took me for a long walk. He taught me how to maneuver on the stairs with my crutches. He encouraged me to try walking with one crutch, but I was not ready. He tried to encourage me to use the hotel swimming pool, as some of the One-Hippers were doing swimming therapy. I was not able to manage the ladder. He taught me how to retrain my walk and not continue with my old gait, which was one that compensated for years of pain. My habit of limping and swinging my left leg outward was to be addressed if I were to walk normally. I now had the mechanics to do so. I remembered reading on the Board about people who struggled to retrain their gait. Those who suffered for many years had a much more difficult time in this process.

Everyday it was necessary for all of us who had surgery to wear the white compression stockings to prevent blood clots. They felt tight and uncomfortable at first. Having someone assist in putting them on in the beginning was a blessing when it was impossible to bend over. They were called TEDS. We were all advised to wear them for five weeks. In the beginning, we wore them day and night. After awhile we had permission from the doctor to remove them to wash them in the evening, putting them back on in the morning. Our compression stockings had open toes and came just above the knee. I remembered reading on the Board about some hippies who were given compression stockings that were from toe to groin and who were to wear them day and night for six weeks after the operation. Different doctors and different situations create different experiences.

In the hospital they taught me to give myself a small injection into the loose skin of my stomach. These injections were to prevent blood clots. I was to do this faithfully for five weeks after surgery. At first I cringed at the thought of it, which caused me to muse that I had just had a major surgery, numerous needles in me, and two large incisions. The comedy was found in the idea of a small needle upsetting me. It did not take long for me to adjust to it and become quite proficient at injecting myself. From the Board I learned that different doctors use different methods to prevent blood clots. Some prescribed oral medications instead of injections. Some doctors supplied their patients with coated aspirin for a five-week period post-op. I thought it would be so much easier to take a pill. My recommendation when it comes to this would be to request a pill and make life easier. Again, different doctors and different situations.

I was not given a lot of medications. The pain was not so strong that I needed it. The naggings created by being so immobile kept me awake at night. I used six pillows under my legs so that my heels would be elevated and not touch the bed. It was the only way I could lay down. The sleeping pills that they gave me after I could not sleep well for four nights did not seem to work. Slowly, everything began to get better.

Daily, for three weeks, I was to administer to myself a strong anti-inflammatory drug in pill form to prevent heterotopic ossification. This condition is caused by the abnormal calcification or ossification of the muscles around the hip joint. 8 It would result in a stiff joint and inhibit normal movement. The symptoms would be pain and a limited range of motion. In severe cases, surgery would have to be performed to remove it. I wanted to prevent this. It is customary for a patient to be put onto medication after a Resurfacing surgery to prevent such problems. This medicine was called Indocid.

It was strange to be so far away from my loved ones and to feel so disabled. I felt a sense of homesickness sweep over me that was very real and very deep. I had just went through a very major surgery. Much to my joy, some of my family members and friends called me and emailed me. D'jango would check my email for me at an Internet cafe. My Mom and my daughters were all praying for me and sending me hugs. My friends also called me to boost my morale. I did not realize how much those phone calls would lift my spirits.

Sixteen

The Second Week post op

It did not take long before I was able to move about more freely. At one-week post surgery, I was in the Holiday Inn next to the hospital. I could get up and walk to the lobby to use the Internet. The food was wonderful in the Holiday Inn restaurant. I felt ravenous. There was a breakfast bar every morning. I attributed huge cravings for fruits, oatmeal, and eggs to being anemic. When I walked into the dining room, I needed to concentrate on each step as well as my posture. I felt like a spectacle, as there were always tourists and business people having a meal or a business meeting. Walking very slowly with my two crutches, and not even having the strength to scoot my chair under the table, seemed to get a lot of glances. After I sat down, D'Jango would slide the table up to me.

I saw my roommate. She had been out of the hospital four days before me. She had already spent nine hours exploring the town of Brugges. She was walking with one cane and did not limp. I watched her walk as though she were a mountain climber ready to take on the Alps. She had her crutch, which seemed to be her mountain climbing staff. She was smiling. Her pants fit her! I was glad that I had taken skirts as I was too swollen to get into my pants! Her hips were level! She was going off onto a new adventure of exploring with her family while I was going to spend much of the day on my back with my legs propped up. My consolation was our nightly excursion of taking a taxi into Ghent where we would dine at one of the many restaurants. After dinner we always returned, as I was exhausted from the outing.

We sometimes shared a meal with fellow Surfacehippies and their families while staying in the hotel. I marveled at how well they walked with one crutch. They would go out sightseeing during the day, of course scheduling their time around when the doctor, the physical therapist, and the nurse would come for the daily visit. They would laugh and share stories of their get-togethers with Belgium beer and chocolates. Having one hip done seemed to me like a breeze. They had far more confidence than I did. Their physical therapy was more complete, I felt, because they could be more active than I was able to be. Their capabilities created more movement and strengthening for the operated side, by having the full use of the unoperated side. I began to wonder if it would have been less healing time to have one hip done at a time, two times, instead of two at one time as I had done. Without any doubt, I knew, despite it all, that I had made the right choice to have both sides done simultaneously. To have the surgery twice would have meant more money spent for plane fares, more time off, but most importantly, having one hip done would not have helped my spinal problem and I definitely wanted to avoid spinal surgery.

In the early weeks after hip surgery, I learned it is much easier to have a bed that is high. This applied to the One-Hippers as well as the Two- Hippers. The beds in the Holiday Inn were low. The low bed made it very difficult to get in and out of bed. I thought about putting a mattress from a hotel roll away or cot on top of my bed to make it higher, but knew that the support I needed for my back would be jeopardized. At this point, I needed to keep my back in check. Difficult as it was, I managed to get in and out of bed with carefully planned and slow movements. I wondered how the taller people managed.

When going out for an evening meal in Ghent, I learned to always take a pillow to sit on, as well as the garbage bag for sliding into the taxi. Of course crutches and a backpack were a necessity, as I did not have free hands to carry a purse.

Every day the nurse came to the hotel room to check on my stitches. On the eleventh day after surgery, he removed them. There was a great deal of sensitivity where the cuts were. He said that my incisions were beautiful.

To my amazement, I realized that I was taller. When looking in the mirror, I thought I seemed to have more stature. I checked my height. Approximately one inch in height was gained from the surgery.

The final meeting with the physical therapist was one of writing down his recommendations for my continuing therapy at home. Dr. Koen De Smet filled the last visit before I left with encouragement and advice. He told me that I could do anything I wanted, but to use common sense. He said that it would be difficult to dislocate my hips. The last day was one of preparing to leave Belgium. Medical travel papers, stating that I could travel, were prepared by my doctor, as well as paperwork showing pictures and explanations of the devices that were implanted in me. I would need these at the airport.

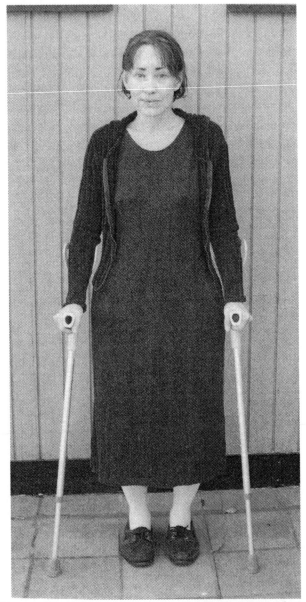

Photo of Peggy two weeks after double hip Resurfacing

Seventeen

There's No Place Like Home

The time for our early morning departure from the Holiday Inn arrived. While some of my One-Hipper friends were driving to Paris for a holiday, I crutched slowly and got my belongings together. We took a taxi from the Holiday Inn in Ghent to the airport in Brussels. The sun rose while we traveled. I did some more sightseeing from the window of the taxi. The farms were lovely. I knew I was in the beginning of a newfound life without pain.

When we arrived at the airport in Brussels, the taxi driver ran to get me a wheelchair. The officials of the airport examined my medical papers. All was well. A woman gently felt over me to make sure I was not carrying bombs or weapons. They were all very kind. We boarded a small plane and flew to London.

In London I felt as though they treated us like royalty. We exited the rear of the plane while everyone else went forward. We went onto a platform, which was lowered slowly, and I was helped onto a wheelchair and wheeled into a van. We were driven to a point where an airport employee took over pushing the wheelchair and took us directly through customs without any hassles. The official examined my paperwork. Then there was a problem. It seemed that the Dallas Texas airport did not recognize something in the paperwork and was concerned that I was not well enough to travel. It took over an hour to straighten it out. The doctor was in surgery and could not be reached. For a while I was faced with having to sleep over in London until the doctor could rewrite the letter. Finally, everything worked out and we were taken onto the plane. The compassion of the Brits still stays with me.

The instructions given to me by my doctor to walk frequently during the flight to prevent blood clots were taken very seriously. Upgrading to business class was well worth the added expense. With crutches and the need to recline, the added space was very useful. The stewardess was there to help me whenever I dropped something or needed help.

When we arrived in Dallas, we had to wait until a wheelchair was brought to the plane. My hips were very swollen and I had to painfully squeeze my hips against the sides of the wheelchair. I would recommend for anyone in this position to request a larger wheel chair. D'Jango pushed me through the airport while I carried my crutches and my backpack. When going through customs, the person checking me took my crutches from me and asked me to stand up. I told her that I had just had double hip surgery and needed my crutches to stand. She allowed me to remain in the chair, but she frisked me in a very rough manner. I was too tired to make a big deal out of it. If I were to give myself advise now, I would have asked her for her name and reported her so that she could be retrained in the proper manner.

Eighteen

The Third Through the Eighth week post op

Knowing that my healing would accelerate in my home was a good feeling. It was so good to be on my own turf. At three weeks post op, I found that using the "reacher" was a vital part of my day as I seemed to drop things often. I carried a backpack around the house with items I wanted to carry from one place to another, since I was still on two crutches and did not have a free hand. I was glad that I had prepared ahead of time and found pots and pans, towels, and washcloths within my reach. Cooking basic meals was not hard with two crutches because I could stand in one place without the crutches. Using the idea of sliding the bar stool to transport items across the kitchen was ingenuous.

Everyday I needed assistance in putting on my TEDs, as my inability to reach my toes affected much of my independence. I always looked forward to taking them off before I went to sleep at night, as they were uncomfortable and inhibited a good rest.

Reading the posts everyday was an aid, as I did not have a physical therapist. Encouraging words always inspired me with the idea of not being in competition in the healing process. To compare oneself to others would be futile, as each of us has a different situation. The words that I always used with my Pilates students, "Never force yourself, just do the best you can do, and you will only get better" were now in my thoughts daily. In the book *Prepare Yourself For Surgery, Heal Faster,* the same idea was expressed in different words. "It is a peaceful sense of surrender that allows healing, rather than commanding it."

Often, I would listen to a tape that I created, in which I visualized myself running through a meadow, lifting my knees high, and feeling my hair blow in the breeze. I visualized coming to a hill, on which I would easily run up, raising my knees high, without any pain. I used

91

some of my favorite music for the background sound on this tape. It helped me a great deal when I was feeling depressed. During week three I did not do my exercises faithfully, as I was so very tired from the trip home. I could not sit for long and I had trouble laying down for the entire night. The encouragement from the Surfacehippies helped me a great deal.

By four weeks post op, I figured a way to put my TEDs on. Using the recliner, I was able to lay back and this created the possibility of slowly bending forward toward my feet. Even though Dr. De Smet told me that it would be very difficult to have a dislocation, I used great caution. Nothing hurt, or seemed to feel forced.

At that time, I was concentrating on specific daily exercises. Taking walks and keeping up with any activities that the physical therapist in Belgium had recommended to me were all I could do. Feelings of fatigue may have been enhanced by possible anemia. Week four brought on other little victories, such as the ability to sit on the toilet. I never did get a raised toilet seat. I also could walk with one crutch indoors and my ability to walk increased to one half of a mile. Using my knowledge of the Pilates exercise system was one of the best things I did for myself. Minimal but precise movements, while concentrating on the specific muscles, were the beginning of a wonderful recovery. Pain was diminishing and I could sleep, even though I could still sleep only on my back. The swelling went down a lot during the fourth week and I could now wear my baggy pants. Massage therapy from my daughter and from D'jango helped me a great deal. I would highly recommend massage, but first you need to get an approval from your doctor. Deep tissue body massage too soon was not advisable according to my doctor.

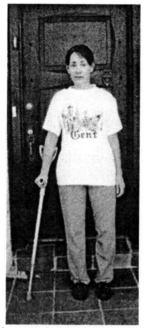

Peggy at five weeks post op using one crutch

By week five I was moving much better. I could move in dancing motion without my crutch. This became a part of my therapy exercises. I would lift my knees and move my body, within reason, using music. I felt wonderful. When reading posts from those who had surgery in America, I realized that they were not doing as much and their limitations were greater.

By week six, I could bring my knees to my chest in a chair. Sleeping on my back was easier, as I was getting more and more accustomed to it. I still could not lay on my sides. With the inability to sit on the floor for the purpose of yoga, I settled into very gentle yoga postures in a chair. Making minimal yogic type movements slowly increased my mobility. One of my early exercises was simply reaching toward my toes. I was only capable of a tiny movement as my capacity was very diminished, but slowly everything remembered what it was made to do. Regaining mobility with slow and caring movements, loving my body into normalcy, would mean to never force anything.

Naturally, the abilities returned. One by one, I would just notice that I had regained a movement.

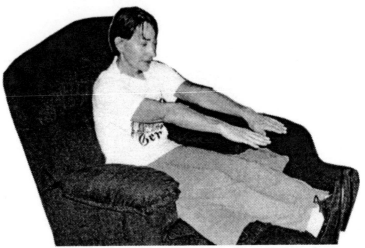

Reaching for the toes with the aid of a reclining chair

By week seven I could lay on my side for thirty minutes. I could go to the grocery store without any crutches and found myself using the shopping cart for support now and then. Stiffness was still a daily occurrence. Concerns arose when my back began to hurt. Of course, the muscles were now being challenged. The Surfacehippies spoke of this problem and described how it takes time for the body has to adjust to its new hips. I could do some gentle squats with my hands on a chair. This relieved the back pain. I felt that I was almost ready to sit on the floor. I could pick things up off the floor by slowly bending over. Every time my abilities increased, I felt a victory.

The process of healing and knowing what to expect could not be measured always by the experience of others, even though the sharing of these experiences was a valuable tool. After all, a set of directions, as you would get with a new camera, did not come with these hips. That is because people are all different in their healing process. My map to recovery was based on the experiences of the hippies, even though I depended on the wisdom of my body to know how far I could push myself.

I spent my eighth week post op following a quest of different sorts. Some of the Surfacehippies on the Board advised against it, but there were a couple, who said that I could do it. I rented a trailer, loaded it with twenty-seven paintings, my display walls, and my tent. With that, I drove for fourteen hours to Louisiana to attend an art exhibit. A friend came with me. I drove the entire way. I felt so excited about my new life. While I drove, I did some energization exercises to keep me from getting too stiff. I would tighten the left thigh, then loosen it. Tighten the right thigh. Then loosen. Then the calves. Then the ankles. Then the feet. Then the back, lower, mid, and upper. The shoulders. The neck. The arms. I read once about a man who developed strong muscles by doing this form of minimal movement exercise. Upon my arrival I was very stiff. I felt as though I was the tin man on the Wizard of Oz. I needed Dorothy and the oil can! A hot bath in the hotel and a good night's rest made all the difference. Eight weeks after double hip surgery, I was sitting in Covington, Louisiana in front of my tent, selling my art. I was dressed in a lovely outfit with a hat and nobody would have suspected. One of the Surfacehippies that I met in the hospital in Ghent happened to live nearby and came to see me. We walked together and compared notes. We shared ideas on healing and regaining our mobility. That trip increased my confidence level immensely.

Nineteen

Week sixteen and my well overflows!

At week sixteen I was walking in the airport. My strides were long and quick. I kept the pace up for a long time. As I realized what I was doing, I began laughing in delight. Did the people around think I was crazy? It did not matter. I could stride! I could strut!

No longer was there pain in my neck! The stiffness that I had developed from years of mechanical problems was still brought to my awareness in the mornings, and could be remedied by yoga stretches. If I had proceeded with a total hip replacement, I would have forfeited these yogic movements that now benefited my life. The lower back, which as I learned has a definite effect on the neck, was working in unison without any surgical fusions! Lifting weights gently and being aware of my developing back muscles became a part of my daily routine. Walking for hours without doing squats became a welcomed possibility. Walking in the shopping mall and walking on the beach were now an amazing new gift. The little things in life, even as simple as sleeping on my sides, became joyous reminders of my blessings. To operate a vacuum cleaner and not feel pain, to delight in walking across the house because I forgot something, to cherish walking the dog filled me with delight. Attending dance lessons and yoga classes weekly brought more thrill to my life. Swimming proved to be one of the finest ways for me to regain muscle strength as well as to have an aerobic workout. The possibility of my returning to my teaching Pilates was becoming a reality.

If I had any type of problem or question an email to my doctor in Belgium would bring me an answer within a day. Dr. De Smet asked that I send to him new X-rays of my hips one year after my surgery.

When I first viewed my scars, I realized that they would always be a reminder of the wonderful people who afforded time and care to make this surgery possible. My scars would also remind me always, of a journey laced with fear and courage to fight for the right of choice. These scars of honor would surely help myself as well as other Surfacehippies to know that we are capable of helping others with the knowledge we have earned, and perhaps, we would consider it to be our duty.

Photos of Peggy six months post op
Yoga poses

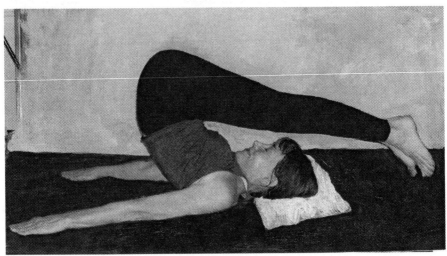

The "plow"

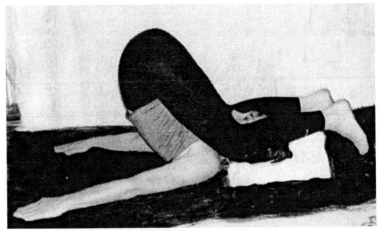

"Knees to ears" pose

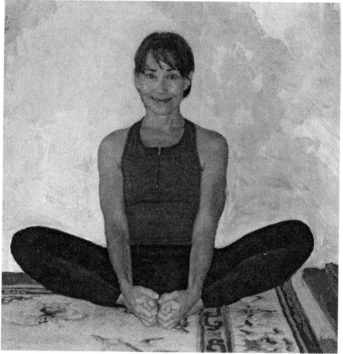

Peggy sitting on the floor

SECTION THREE

CASES AND EXPERIENCES

The story of Edith
Edith is an incredible woman whose pain and victory has inspired many.

Thirty-five years ago, I had my hip fused. This was the final step taken by my Osteopath, who was then treating a serious infection in my left hip. The infection was very septic and lodged in the area of the pelvis. The fusion was carefully and meticulously done, which would ultimately be a very important factor thirty-five years later, when I would go under the knife again.

My fused hip placed huge and very unnatural pressures on almost every joint in my body. The most damage happened to my spine and my knee, as they were forced to take the bending load. Even sitting was an ordeal, as my back had to bend in a most unnatural way. With time, the other joints became arthritic also. My system seemed to be closing down. Personal things such as using the toilet, dressing, and even traveling in a car became more and more difficult. Problems with my spine were ever increasing, and I struggled to cope.

For many years I asked to be given a hip replacement. I was always told that a total hip replacement was not for me, as the shaft that they would have to put down my femur would be too invasive.
The doctors believed that it was possible that a total hip replacement could indeed trigger the return of the infection that I might be prone to. The name of this infection was Osteomyelitis. Another reason that I did not qualify for a total hip replacement was the atrophy of the surrounding hip muscles. They told me that the hip muscles help to prevent the dislocation problems associated with a total hip replacement.

Treatment for my condition was just to keep me out of pain as much as possible. Painkillers were a part of my daily life. I dealt daily with the increasing closure of anything that resembled living a normal life. I was even denied the comfort of retiring to a wheel chair, as by the end of 33 years I could hardly sit any more without severe pain and

103

discomfort. Sitting with a fused hip is not sitting, but more of a manipulation that distorts the body into painful mutations.

I finally resorted to contemplating on how I could talk a surgeon into amputating my leg at the hip, so that I could at least sit in a wheel chair without pain. My ability to walk was not so valuable to me, if I could eliminate the pain.

In March of 2002, another incident occurred which put my back into an even nastier condition. I could not hold my torso upright any longer or walk for several days. My chiropractor, who was always so helpful in the past when my back was so wretched, found it to be more difficult than ever to ease the pain. The spine refused to cooperate. Sitting was impossible.

Instead of just relying on what the contracted doctors said, I decided to go onto the Internet and search for answers. I found the Total Hip List and decided that I had nothing to lose with posing the question whether anyone knew someone in my condition who was able to have a total hip replacement. One woman replied in a few hours. She had a similar experience as mine. She referred me to four OS doctors in the USA and also recommended an article about the undoing of fused hips, and giving them total hip replacements. This information had an effect on me that is indescribable. After dealing with tears, I decided that I would set out to find an OS in Australia who could help me.

Finding an OS who would even talk to me was not easy. My sister, who is a General Practitioner, helped me with the search. One OS told me to go to the US if I knew that this surgery was done there. Others said that because of the Osteomyelitis problems, they could not do it. The local hospital doctors were even less supportive.

Finally the winds began to change for me. My brother-in-law had done the anesthetic for a young OS just out of training in Sydney. He was impressed by this doctor's work and discussed my problem with him. From this discussion, I was led to a doctor in Sydney. This man was the first doctor I had ever spoken with who could explain what was happening to me and why. He told me that he had separated fused bones and followed with a total hip replacement twice before with success. He also said that he was the only one who had done it in Australia. The surgery is difficult and requires that a surgeon chip the fused bones apart before the hip replacement can be performed. I obtained the MRIs, bone scans, and X-rays that he requested. I truly felt that I would have crawled the fifteen hundred miles to Sydney from my home to see him, so strong was my desire to get some relief from my impossible situation.

My appointment with him revealed his concerns about inviting the osteomyelitis bone infection to return with the long shank of the Total hip replacement being driven down into the femur. He knew another route, it was the Birmingham Hip Resurfacing, BHR, device. He explained that the stem is not nearly as intrusive and that the devise does not dislocate easily. The result of this appointment was a surgery date set with this doctor. Now it was time to prepare.

My realization to being as fit and prepared as possible was a key to my recovery time being as easy as possible. I began using a lot of concentration to activate the muscles in my thigh. That gave me the hope that I could find other muscles later.

On the morning of August 2, 2002, I threw the dice and took the consequences. The operation went like a dream. It took only three hours and twenty minutes. There were not any infections. The wound healed well.

That was only one of the many battles I was to face. Now was the question, could I make my leg move under my own control again? The early therapy was exhausting. The leg went into spasms at suddenly finding itself moving again. Slowly, it did respond to my efforts. By day seventeen, I was sent home. I was not bearing any weight on the operated leg and used crutches to get around. Those first few weeks at home were so very difficult.

At six months after the surgery, I could bend my leg to seventy degrees. It was strong enough that I could lift it off of the bed. After thirty-five years of atrophy in my muscles, I found myself swimming almost every day. I know that I will never have totally normal movement because of all of the damage from the years of distorting my back, but I have my life back. No longer am I in a state of becoming more and more isolated and miserable.

After the operation, my skin color became a normal and healthy tone, which it had not been for years. My doctor could not explain it, but I suspect that the lack of normal circulation and movement of muscles over a long period of time played a role. I was told by many people that I appeared to be ten years younger. My appearance was also affected by my being more fit and active. All thanks to a few bits of metal and a wonderful doctor who was prepared to do an operation that would make a difference.

Brenda's Hip Blessing
Brenda, currently a photographer in Texas, was born with an undeveloped hip.

The following document is a letter written by Brenda's mother. The missive, written to Brenda's grandmother, depicts a traumatic experience targeting a Texas family through the ordeal of a small child.

Dear Mama,

April 13, 1958

Well I hardly know where to begin to tell you about Brenda. After she came out of the cast, she took a good while to learn to walk again but bless her heart, she did. However, she limped so badly that she fell quite a bit. Then in February I took her for a check & x-rays were made and then he told me the news. Her hip socket still was not formed enough and the leg bone was pushed up beyond the socket. She would have to go back to the hospital and be put in traction, have the cast put back on and then have two operations. I can't tell you how it shocked us both – I went around in a daze to think that little girl had to go through all that again – and even more this time – but she's a trooper and she has a spirit that can't fail. And I believe God can do anything and C.B. and I have the faith that He is going to make Brenda well so she can run with the rest. Just remember her in your prayers because I know she is going to have fine straight legs in the near future.

Love to All,
-Danelle

Brenda remembers how it was to be a child experiencing several hip surgeries. At thirteen months of age, it was discovered that she had hip dysplasia. Her undeveloped hip socket, which compromised the femur, had made the simple act of learning to walk a real challenge. Her unusual first years of life brought the experience of a body cast to a baby who was hardly more than one year of age. The cast had to be removed several times over a period of two years, as the child was outgrowing the plaster cocoon that encased her from just below her breasts to her toes. She could not sit. Her father fashioned a paddleboard with castor wheels for her, so she could use her arms scoot around the floor face down on her belly. Her mother would often put her plate onto the floor and little Brenda would pull herself up to it for a meal.

"The abundant love and caring that my mother gave me helped me get through a very difficult experience. One of my memories was of my mother lovingly sitting a plate of hot biscuits down onto the floor for me one morning, with the sun streaming through the windows making patterns of light on the floor for me to roll my scooter through."

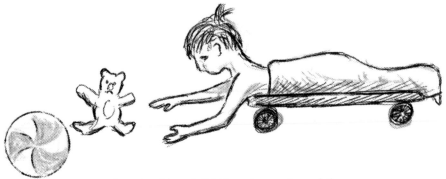

Sketch of the child-Brenda at play while
encased in the plaster cocoon

"I remember the feeling of being a small child trapped inside of a plaster prison, calling out at night for my mother to come and turn me over when I became restless with not being able to move."

She was heavy. Her mother became pregnant again and it was difficult to lift the small child with the heavy cast.

The surgeon who gave Brenda a normal childhood took a piece of the small child's hip bone and grafted it into place to help form a socket. By the time Brenda was old enough to start school, she was able to walk and even run and play. Throughout elementary school she was a runner and competed in the athletic events of her school. She limped, but did not consider it to be a hindrance.
"I never was conscious of an actual limp; it was more like walking differently from the others".

In high school, when she naturally wanted to be like the other girls, she became more aware of her different way of walking. In college she still limped, but still, she thought that the problem had been overcome. She never suspected that she would ever need to have hip surgery again, until she began to have some hip pain as a young woman. It was then that a doctor told her that eventually she would need to have a total hip replacement.

By the time Brenda reached her forties, the pain was beginning to increase. It was becoming so intense that she was beginning to consider the surgery. As she learned about the surgery, and the limitations that came with it, she was hesitant.

Brenda wished there were other options. It seemed that there were none. But finally, the option of Resurfacing was brought to the light. By doing some of her own research, she obtained the names of some doctors who did the Resurfacing technique. Mailing X-rays always led to the same thing, a doctor who did not think that she was a candidate for a Resurfacing. The structure of her hip was very worn and the bone was somewhat soft. Every doctor who viewed her X-rays said that the abnormal shape of the pelvis and the lack of a sufficient socket would make it a complicated procedure that only a total hip replacement could remedy.

Her next step was to mail her X-rays to the doctor in Belgium, as she had heard a great deal about him. His response was that he could do the Resurfacing surgery.

Once again, Brenda's mother wanted to help her daughter. Brenda's brother also wanted to help. The trio flew to Belgium together.

Her surgery went normally, but her recovery was a little longer than many of the other one hippers, due to the softer bone.
Her life is totally different now since she can walk for miles without pain. She can dance without pain. Her life is one that no longer requires pain pills. She is practicing yoga and is enjoying many activities that she could not do before.
"To wake up every morning and know that I can expect an active and pain free day, without medications, is a blessing for which I am ever so grateful!"

"Dancer of the year" the story of Maya

My name is Maya, and I am a Surfacehippy. I am 47 years old and had a very long and active career as a professional modern dancer and choreographer. I began dancing at a relatively late age, 17, but made up for lost time and managed to get into a professional company right out of college. My training included extensive ballet and modern with some jazz and tap. The training was rigorous. I taught and rehearsed dance until I was 39. When I performed, I did not know how hard it was on my hips. Sometimes, I would perform works that would last over an hour and never leave the stage. I was known for my high leg extensions, deep lunges, and dramatic performances. I actually won some awards in Chicago and was voted by my peers as "Dancer of the Year."

The pain in my hip did not start until I was 36. I remember being in a dance class where the teacher based every exercise on the psoas muscle, which included lots of leg lifting and holding the leg in the air for a long time. At one point, my leg dropped to the floor and I couldn't walk for three days. That was the beginning of the end. I had burning pain in my hip for the next six years. I managed to keep dancing professionally for a few more years until I became pregnant at 39. I stopped dancing for a year and that's when the arthritis set in. By the time I was 40, I was told that it was time for a hip replacement.

As the performing career was winding down, I began to teach Pilates. I found that I enjoyed it and it kept me from getting that hip replacement for another six years. I could not hike, ride a bike, or tie my shoe. I had to drag my leg into my car. After working with clients who had total hip replacements, I decided that was not for me. They had such limited range of motion and either kept dislocating their hips (not in my class) or had fears of dislocation.

Finally, a fellow Pilates teacher told me about a client of hers who had a new type of hip surgery. **When I learned about the concept**

of hip Resurfacing, I knew that I wanted it: full range of motion without cutting off the ball of my hip.

I called her client, who told me about another dancer, William Starrett, who had both hips done. I spoke with William and saw a video of him performing with his resurfaced hips. I called his surgeon immediately. It did not take long to discover that my insurance policy would not cover this surgery. My husband and I took out a loan on our house to pay for the surgery. The surgery changed my life. I am dancing on two legs again, chasing after my seven-year old, and free of pain. It is miraculous.

The Athlete With Two Naughty Hips
Saeed's passion for his sport brought him to the discovery of Hip Resurfacing

In 1988, I was doing some hill running for training. It was then that I started to notice some muscle pain in the front of the left thigh. It began to bother me on the tennis court whenever I made a quick move. Thinking of it as just a bad pull, I did not go to a doctor until the following September. The pain actually went away for much of the summer.

When I finally saw the doctors, they had trouble seeing anything on the X-rays at first. They thought I might have AVN for use of prednisone for a past dermatology prescription. They eventually spotted Osteoarthritis on the X-rays and predicted that my right hip would probably mimic the left in the process of deterioration. It took two years to see that their prediction was correct.

I cannot begin to describe how I felt about having a hip problem. I had just become the state of Wisconsin's champion in tennis for the age 35 category. Possibly, I was on my way to become nationally ranked. I was improving with age and maintained my youthfulness and athletic abilities. All of sudden, my orthopedic doctor was looking at my X-rays and telling me that I had the hips of a 65 -year old!

In an attempt to develop a positive attitude and change my life style from one of athletic development, I looked to do something more productive in the business or education world. This did not eliminate the physical pain or the depression from loosing something I loved. The reality was that it changed my life to a struggle of maintaining a positive attitude. Regardless, I did the best I could to maintain hope that through exercise and diet, I would maintain myself and hope for medical breakthroughs.

Continuing to play tennis on a more limited schedule only reminded me of the stiffness and pain that accompanies Osteoarthritis. For the next thirteen years, my condition slowly worsened. I could never regain my range of motion, not to mention my ability to sustain running or quick movements. I worked at improving some of my tennis skills in the hand and mind aspects.

I knew that I wanted to avoid having a total hip replacement at all costs, even though my friends and family sometimes encouraged it. My doctor told me that once I had a THR, I would never be able to run or play any tennis effectively without endangering the longevity of the prosthesis. The pains in my hip began to grow more serious. There were some new pains in the gluteal area. I was sure that my condition was worsening.

While researching on the Internet for information about the THR, I found the link to the Birmingham site on hip Resurfacing.

I was thrilled to read about the testimonials of athletes and what they could do after surgery. I could instantly see that the procedure and the device made so much sense and how vastly superior the whole method seemed. My life changed on that day.

After months of failing at being approved by my insurance company for the Resurfacing surgery in the United States, I decided to go to Europe for a double BHR. It was the best thing I could have done. Having two hips done at the same time was very difficult, but with patience in my healing process, the fruits of my labor arrived. To regain my movement, my youth, and my love for tennis is an unimaginable blessing. I also get a lot of satisfaction in helping others discover this marvelous new surgery.

Questions to Dr. De Smet:

Question: What are the most common causes of failure in a total hip replacement?

Dr. De Smet: **Osteolysis and loosening caused by Polyethylene wear is the most common cause of failure in a total hip replacement. Another cause is from a poor technique by the surgeon, bad positioning of the implant, recurrent dislocation and infections.**

Question: Where is the pain localized when I suffer from Osteoarthritis?

Dr. De Smet: **Pain is mostly localized in the groin, buttock region, but can also refer to the whole thigh, lumbar and even the knee.**

Question: How long does an average total hip replacement last?

Dr. De Smet: **This depends on the age, activity of the patient, and of course the implant itself!**

Question: Do you believe that a Resurfacing will outlast the total hip replacement and why?

Dr. De Smet: **Resurfacing will out last a THR, and certainly in young patients, because of the use of MOM (metal on metal) which has the capacity of low wear and the CONSERVATION OF BONE. Unless there are contra-indications, which are osteoporosis, deformed femoral head, or a bad technique by the surgeon, there would be very few reasons why a Resurfacing would not outlast a THR.**

Question: Are there a greater amount of problems when you operate on two hips at the same time?

Dr. De Smet: In severe osteoarthritis of both hips, a bilateral procedure can be done. Both hips are opened up on the same day. Our experience today has not given more problems when this is performed on healthy patients. A continous epidural catheter and more blood transfusions are needed.

Question: If there were a revision for Resurfacing, could another Resurface be done?

Dr. De Smet: I did a revision of a Resurfacing with a Resurfacing, but at this point in time, I think a classical Total Hip Replacement will be done. In the future, this can always change.

Question: Do you think that patients should be concerned about metal ions in the blood?

Dr. De Smet: No, I do not. Do you realize that if you drink a beer there are metal ions also coming into the bloodstream? With all of the studies done today, I am convinced that metal ions in the blood stream should not raise any concerns.

Question: Are the metal ions in the blood from a BHR metal on metal device greater, the same, or less than from a metal on metal THR?

This is still under investigation. I am conducting my own studies on this. I do not think that the metal ions in the Resurfacing or THR will differ that much. I believe that the types of metals will be the factor. With the big ball in Resurfacing, we know that the lubrication in between both

components can be thicker than in the THR because of the difference in diameter. On the other hand, the bigger surface can possibly create more corrosion, even if there is no wearing of the prosthesis.

Question: Is Resurfacing for large boned as well as small boned people? Do the devices come in various sizes?

Yes, the devices do come in various sizes. For every measure of patient, there is a measure of prosthesis. The art is to match the correct size of the prosthesis to the hip.

Question: Please explain about the possibility of palsy of the femoral nerve as a result of hip surgery.

Dr. De Smet: With a femoral nerve palsy it is difficult to walk because the quadriceps do not work. The patient will not be able to keep the leg extended while walking. This normally disappears spontaneously. Even though this seldom happens, there is less chance of it happening with a BHR than a THR. The posterior approach is a factor that lessens the risk of femoral nerve palsy, but the possibility of having the Ischial nerve elongated or cut could result in pain and dysfunction of the muscles and nerves.

Question: What if a woman becomes pregnant after she receives a hip Resurfacing?

Dr. De Smet: Research has proven that the metal ions do not go through the placenta. To become pregnant and have children after hip surgery is very possible without problems.

Question: If I have a hip prosthesis, and I become ill with a bad cold and laryngitis, do I need to be on antibiotics to protect my new hip?

Dr. De Smet: Colds are viruses and antibiotics will not have any effect on them. Antibiotics need to be taken only for bacterial infections.

Question: Do you think it would be safe for a patient to travel in a third world country where there could be higher risks to disease and infections?

Dr. De Smet: I do not believe that there would be any more risk than anyone else. Traveling with antibiotics would be a good idea, but it is important to make sure an entire dosage for one or two weeks would be carried, as antibiotics in short bursts can cause bacteria that is resistant to the antibiotics. I do not believe that this is a major concern.

Question: Is it true that people who have an artificial hip prosthesis need to take certain precautions when going to the dentist?

Dr. De Smet: I advise my patients to have an antibiotic prescribed to them to take preceding dental treatments to eliminate possibilities of bacterial infections.

Question: Is it possible to fracture neck of the femur during a BHR surgery?

Dr. De Smet: This is possible, but should not happen. This is the worst complication that I am aware of with this surgery. In the unlikelihood of this happening, the patient can be given the Resurfacing cup with a stem and a big modular head. This would give an

**excellent range of movement with very low risk of
dislocations in comparison with a classical hip
replacement prosthesis.**

Question: Does being overweight significantly interfere with the
               hip Resurfacing surgery?

**Dr. De Smet: Resurfacing surgery can be performed on
overweight people, even though it may be less than
ideal. There will be other precautions to consider
also. Surgery under this condition is more difficult.**

Question: Is it safe for a hip Resurfacing patient to receive an
               ultrasound?

**Dr. Koen De Smet: Ultrasound done at the hip area of a metal
on metal prosthesis can heat up and burn the bone.**

Question: During surgery when you use the posterior approach,
               are muscles cut?

**Dr. Koen De Smet: The muscles that are cut and reattached
during the posterior approach are the external
rotators.**

Question: What is the name of the other approach that can be
               used for this surgery, and why don't you use it?

**Dr. Koen De Smet: The other approach often used is lateral or
anterolateral approach which ALWAYS damages
the abductor muscles, which are the glutaeus
medius muscle. This can result in problems with
the gait. The cutting of these muscles also inhibits
quick recovery. I used this approach in my first
1200 prosthesis, half or more of the surgeons are
still using this approach as they are concerned**

about dislocations with the posterior approach. I, also, do not use the lateral approach because of the unanatomical approach and problems with bursitis.

Question: What was the age of the youngest patient whom you resurfaced? What was the age of the oldest patient?

Dr. Koen De Smet: The youngest child was fourteen-years old, and very disabled. That child returned to a normal life. The oldest patient was seventy-six years old.

Question: What are the most frequent complications that a patient can experience after having hip surgery?

Dr. Koen De Smet: The most encountered complications are:

Deep Vein Thrombosis (DVT) and Pulmonary Embolis (PE). Post-operative DVT is one of the most common complications following hip or knee surgery. This condition can occur in up to fifty percent of patients and often, there are no symptoms. It is caused by the damage done to the veins during the surgery in combination with immobilization.

Pulmonary embolus (PE) is when a blood clot is formed and travels to the lung. It occurs only three per cent of the time and can be sudden and fatal. We take several measures to prevent the formation of clots in the legs. Compression stockings are worn by the patient day and night while in the hospital. In addition, there are exercises that the patient can do in bed, as well as drugs to thin the blood.

Dislocation is another possible complication. It happens when the ball of the hip joint comes out of

the socket. This problem is preventable by patient education and care. Chances of dislocation after a total hip replacement are 1%, increasing to 10% after total hip revision surgery. The BHR hip Resurfacing procedure has an extremely low dislocation rate, and actually, we have not seen any dislocations at all!

Nerve Injury:
Whenever an incision is made, it is possible to damage the sensory nerves in that area. This type of injury, which is not very common, can occur while lengthening the hip more than one inch. A congenital hip deformity or revision total hip replacement would be more at risk for this. Nerve injuries of this type can result in the patient not being able to raise the ankle or toe. This is called 'foot drop' and is from damage to the Ischial Nerve. In the possibility of palsy of the Femoral Nerve, the patient will not be able to keep the leg extended while walking. This normally disappears spontaneously.

Fracture of the shaft (femur)
This can happen during a total hip replacement or a revision for a total hip replacement when bringing in the prosthesis. It is usually due to osteoporosis or bone loss, or in case of revision surgery, osteolysis. We have proven ways to cope with this problem.

Infection:
The incidence of infection is 1% overall. It can occur as late as a year after surgery. If it is treated early, antibiotics are used and re-operation to clean out the hip. The goal is to attempt to save the prosthesis from removal. Late infection most often

requires re-operation, removal of the prosthesis, intravenous antibiotics, and the possibility of re-implanting the prosthesis when it is safe and the infection it gone.

Question: Is the possibility to have a drop foot occur more frequent with a THR than with a BHR?

Dr. De Smet: Drop foot is a problem of sciatic nerve palsy. This is when a nerve is damaged during the posterior approach in either the THR or the BHR. I do not see this often.

Question: What is your greatest success story with BHR?

Dr. De Smet: Half marathon runner, champion tennis player, heavy sea windsurfer, Mont Blanc and Kilimanjaro climber, Triatlon runner, competition paraglider. Everyday people are amazing me. But the greatest successes are just the happiest people, whatever they do!

Question: How old is the BHR procedure?

Dr. De Smet: The BHR procedure is 6 years old. The metal-on-metal resurfacing is 11 years old.

Posts From The Board

NOTE: The following excerpts are taken from the Surfacehippy site. These posts do not necessarily represent all situations or facts. They were chosen by the author to help increase the understanding of the reader.

Hip Resurfacing failures

Planmaster@yahoo.com

We need to be aware of what brought all of us to this discussion group in the first place. It was the failure of our "native" hip surfaces. If there was one correct answer, we would not see so many disagreements about treatment and types of surgery.

The metal on metal hip Resurfacing technique is obviously an excellent choice for many people. Since we all face the risk that the resurfaced hip will fail, we also realize there is not a lot we can do to prevent it.

Something we can do is to have a bone densitometry exam of both hips and the lumbar spine before surgery. If one hip has been operated on, check the other side. If you have osteoporosis, a THR will be necessary.

If you have osteoporosis, there are effective treatments. The bottom line is to prevent this bone deteriorating disease.

Driving after surgery

Dusthip@wmich.edu

I started driving on the seventh day after surgery. The hardest part was getting in and out of the car. Be careful. One crutch on day fourteen, no crutch or cane by week three. The hip gets better every day!

Beartcke@anabaptists.org

Since I was not expressly forbidden to do so, I tried out driving our minivan at eight days after my conserve plus operation. Fortunately, the operation was on the left hip, which did not have anything to do during the drive. If it had been on the right hip, it would have been a different story, since the operated side would have had to at least press the accelerator.

Eleven days after surgery
ebicth@smartchat.net.au

I am eleven days post op and would like to tell you how I am doing. I had my left hip resurfaced with the Birmingham hip Resurfacing device. I walk with a stick for half an hour each morning and twice for fifteen minutes later in the day.

I do my physio exercises three or four times a day.

I experience stiffness when I sit or lay for any length of time. My staples come out tomorrow. The hardest exercise that I do is lifting my leg onto a step that is about eight inches high while keeping my pelvis straight. The most difficult part of walking is to bring my left leg straight through on each step. For the past year, I have always swung my leg out to the left. It feels great to be able to stand up straight with equal weight on both legs.

Twelve days after surgery
Veenise@nssmgmt.com

I was resurfed twelve days ago in Belgium. I just got home. It was a heck of a trip, but the main thing is that the surgery went well. I am getting along nicely on one crutch. I can actually get around the house without crutches! I am not taking any pain medicine, but I am still taking the indomethacin to prevent heterotopic bone growth. The discomfort is minimal. If I had to do it over again, I would come to Belgium and stay for at least a week to get over the jet lag and tiredness before the surgery. I had the surgery on my second day there. I had a 16 or 20 tough hours after the surgery. I have never had major surgery before and it was tough when the anesthesia wore off and I had to keep my right leg extended. I am a restless sleeper and craved being able to turn onto my side. Nausea also was not any fun. It was all tolerable and the situation improved rapidly. The next day, when my roommate and I were encouraged to get up and use our walkers, everything changed. After that it was time to use the crutches. When learning about my surgery, I discovered that it was possible that I would have awakened with a total hip replacement if I had seen a more conservative doctor. All in all, I am very pleased.

Gait analysis
Treeni@aol.com
Apparently many of you are hoping to have your walks analyzed, and I am sure that a qualified PT/kinesiologist could do a fairly good eyeball assessment.
What we are talking about is a Gait Analysis Laboratory. Check to see if there is one near you. I've been instructed to wear tight-fitting bike shorts, since they will be gluing "markers" to my legs/hips and then digitally photographing and computer mapping the way I walk. The whole process takes over two hours. The fellow who runs the lab watched me walk and could see that my strides were not even. He said I needed more strength in my left leg.
I am sure other places have this technology!

Can Surfers ever have MRIs again?
Mymds@triad.rr.com
I am a radiologist, using MRI daily.
The Resurfacing implants are safe with any MRI examination. Some orthopedic devices cause artifacts which interfere with the quality of some of the MRI images. Common examples are plates and screws used in some types of spinal fusion.

These same devices cause artifacts which degrade the quality of Ct exams because of scattering of the X-ray beam. The newer scanners can overcome this with thinner imaging slices and improved processing software.
To sum it up, MRIs are not dangerous to you. There is nothing left to examine on an MRI of the hips. MRI of the lumbar spine is more limited in the lower area, otherwise no problem. The MRI will not damage the Resurfacing devices.

Hip squeaks like a rusty gate
Samkinc@aol.com
My Cormet 2000 seems to be very noisy sometimes when I put a lot of weight on my operated leg.
The squeaking, as I understand, is pretty normal for up to one year or more and should decline with time. It is probably just part of the

normal wear-in process. During the first month, my hips made noise very frequently when walking. I am now one year and eight months post op, and still get the occasional noise, usually when I am breaking new ground in my range of motion.

Clunking and noises from the prosthesis
Strow@yahoo.com

Hi, I have a BHR…and yes, it does clunk! My muscles were nonexistent after many years of atrophy. The sound has gradually lessened to barely noticeable at six months post op. I suspect that muscle operation and tightness is a major component in this situation. I still notice it after swimming a couple of laps and, even then, it is decreasing rapidly with each swim session.

Siltno1@mindspring.com

I am eleven months out from a Conserve plus Resurfacing in the left hip and still, occasionally, get what feels like a clunk. Keep in mind that my joints were significantly traumatized during the operation and a lot of stuff was pulled and pushed out of place to allow the surgeon access. In addition, there are the physical differences of having the added prosthesis to the joint area.

Exercise after surgery
Dankey@hotmail.com

I was on crutches for six weeks after surgery, as I had a high fracture risk. However, my physical therapist gave me exercises to do laying on the bed from day one and a couple standing on my good leg, but bending and stretching the operated one (from about day 4 or 5).

With some of the bed exercises, your movements can be tiny, but each day the movement becomes easier and your muscles get stronger (from little acorns, as they say)!

Today I just had my second hydrotherapy session (seven weeks post op) and my physical therapist says that I am trying to do too much too soon. She is insisting that it will definitely do more harm than good and will only hold up progress if I try to push myself too hard.

As other people have said on this Board, in the whole scheme of things, what is another couple of weeks going to matter as long as we get there in the end? It is frustrating, yes, but the important thing is to do things correctly and I'd rather take things slowly now and get it totally right than put myself back a couple of months and perhaps damage something permanently.

I think there is a risk that we read some of the posts where people are cycling, going to the gym, and doing all sorts of energetic things within a matter of weeks and we think we should be able to do it also. I know I am guilty of this and start to think that there is something wrong with me. I am beginning to realize that this is not how it works.

I am sure that for some of the younger amongst us who were extremely fit and active post op, quicker recoveries and more vigorous exercise regimes are possible, but, again, I think this is where we all have to look at our individual situations and listen to our own bodies.

It seems obvious that our backgrounds play a huge role in our recovery times. This hip is a new beginning for me and I really want to make it work. I am thus going to have to slow down to achieve this!

Pilates exercises and Rehab
Peggathy@aol.com

Those of us who spent years having our muscles and ligaments restricted, perhaps due to the defective joints, will have to spend a long time re-educating them. Those of us who have a well developed muscle memory of stretching and moving the muscles will surely recover more rapidly. Thus, it is a wise choice to exercise before surgery. Being a Pilates instructor, I know from experience that the Pilates exercises are controlled and safe. They are ideal for people rehabilitating from an accident as well as surgery. The early exercises after surgery are locating the weak muscles. Using precise minimal movements with concentration and focus on specific muscles, without endless repetitions and momentum keep it safe. Gently challenging the muscles in the beginning in the most minimal way is very effective. The muscles respond, and thus become stronger a little at a time. Joseph Pilates, who developed this exercise system, used to say that it is the mind itself that builds the body.

Avascular Necrosis (AVN)
Powman107@yahoo.com

The blood supply to my left hip joint was cut off. If they would have caught it early enough, they could have drilled a hole in the femoral head to get the blood supply to the joint. I was lucky that it was not so advanced, as I was still eligible for a Resurfacing. The pain was immense. At the end, I could not figure out if the pain was due to the AVN or osteoarthritis. I still do not know how long I had AVN. My GP was not much help and told me to take ibuprophen. It took about six 7.5 vicodins a day to take the edge off. He thought it was the osteoarthritis, which I had for ten years starting with small twinges of pain on occasion escalating to extreme throbbing with no relief at the end. Life is wonderful now!

A Big Scare
Slimrunner@ yahoo.com

Two weeks after my Resurfacing arthroplasty, my incision started to get red and warm. I went to the ER and consulted with an OS there. They gave me blood tests and urged me to have surgery the following day, as they were convinced that I had a hip infection, and that two weeks out of surgery is the time. He said that I would have to have two surgeries, one to remove the prosthesis that was currently in my hip and another, later, putting another in after the infection was gone. I realized that I had no fever. I had no hip pain out of the ordinary. I wanted antibiotics and to go home. I said that I would rather be in California near the hip surgeon if it came to surgery.

When I finally was able to reach my hip surgeon, he said that he believes that it was a fat necrosis which was causing the redness and warmth. As long as there was not any fever or pain, it was not likely to be a problem, he reassured me. I am continuing the antibiotics anyway, for the duration.

Metal Detectors at Airports
Trapad@aol.com

Metal detectors at airports do not always detect that I have metal in my hips. I went through one in Houston recently and it did not go off.

I was told by an employee at another airport that the person who leads their training sessions has a metal hip prosthesis and does not make the metal detector react. It may be much simpler and perhaps wiser to not go through the metal detector and to tell them that you are carrying metal. I do not even think the paperwork or card showing that you have a prosthesis is necessary, as anyone could create one it seems. They will put you through a painless search with hand held metal detectors and you will probably have to take off your shoes.

Sound Advise For After Surgery
Samimes @ aol.com

I recently bought a kitchen appliance that comes nicely packaged in a box with a full set of instructions in several languages. I mused at the idea that I did not get my set of instructions with my new hips. Yet, what I know I shall share with you:

Be aware of any possible infections in your body. Do not wait for something that you think may be an infection to get worse.

Precautions need to be taken every time you go to a dentist. Before any dental procedures are done, you will need to take a recommended dose of an antibiotic to prevent infection. Avoid ultrasound in the area of the hips. Develop an awareness for your body and never push anything or force anything.

If you are taking a multi-vitamin, it may be a good idea consider checking it to see if it contains chromium. If it does, you can replace it with a multi-vitamin that does not have chromium.

References Cited

1. http://whitaker.org/glance/hipjoint.html
2. http://whitaker.org/glance/hipjoint.html
3. www.medscape.com
4. www.activejoints.com/bhr_Brochure.pdf
5. www.hip-int.com

Internet
Sources of Information

Surfacehippy message Board
http://groups.yahoo.com/group/surfacehippy

Dr. De Smets website
http://www.hip-clinic.com
http://www.hip-clinic.com/en/html/answers.shtml

Heterotopic Ossification
www.orthoteers.co.uk/nrujpnij33lm/orththrho.html

To see an animation on Resurfacing
http://www.hipResurfacing.com.au/hipResurfacing/

For an interesting article on Birmingham Hip Replacement
http://www.medscape.com/viewarticle/412561

To increase your understanding about the Birmingham Resurfacing
system, and the differences between Resurfacing and the total hip
replacement, you can go to
www.midmedtec.co.uk.co.

To see actual photos of the surgical procedure go to
http://imagesthunderballhip

For great information on hip surgery
http://www.activejoints.com/surgery.html

Blue Cross Blue Shield health insurance company description of Hip Resurfacing:
http://medpolicy.bluecrossca.com/policies/surgery/hip_re

For names of doctors that use the Conserve plus
http://activejoints.com/hipdocs.html

Joint disorders information
http://hipuniverse.homestead.com

Hip implant and surgery research, implant manufacturers, dental precautions, Total Hip Replacements
www.http//hipuniverse.homestead.com/hipurls.html

Totally Hip Discussion Board, owned and maintained by Linda May-Bower; for personal stories about total hip replacements
http://members.tripod.com/totally hip1/

To see hip surgery animations
http://swarminteractive.com/orthopedic/interactive

This site provides valuable information from the South Carolina Joint Replacement Center.
http://www.grossortho.com/education.html

Good information, plenty of good links
http://www.hipsurgery.com.au/hipreplacement/index.htm

Duke Total Joint Center
http://dukehealth.org/ortho/total_joint_hip_Resurfacing.asp

Other Sources of Information

Heal Your Hips by Robert Klapper, M.D. and Lynda Huey

Prepare for Surgery, Heal Faster by Peggy Huddleston

Some Hip Resurfacing Doctors listed below:

Europe:

Dr. Koen De Smet
Heupspecialist
Kalverbosstraat 31a
9070 Heusden Belgium
0032(0)26457
www.hipclinic.com
Koen.desmet@skynet.be

Dr. Derek McMinn
UK telephone: 121 455 0411
Royal Orthopaedic Hospital
Birmingham Nuffield Hospital
Derek.mcminn@ic24.net
http://www.specialistinfo.com/data/consget.php?con=mcmiortp01

List of Some of the Conserve Plus Participating Surgeons In the U.S.

California
Dr. Harlan Amstutz, Dr. Thomas Schmalzried, and Dr. Paul Beaule
Joint Replacement Institute, Los Angeles Orthopaedic Hospital
213-742-1075

Vancouver, WA
Dr. Ed Sparling
360-254-6161

Salem, OR
Dr. Harold Boyd
503-581-4402

Texas, Galveston
Dr. Mike Grecula
Univ. Of Texas Medical Branch
409-772-2565

Sarasota, Florida
Dr. William Kennedy
941-365-0655

Baltimore, MD
Dr. Michael Mont
410-601-8500

Durham, NC
Dr. Tom Vail, Duke Univ.
919-684-4007

List of Some of the Cormet 2000 Participating Surgeons

Colombia, SC
Dr. Tom Gross
803-256-4107

Baltimore, MD
Dr. Michael Jacobs
410-532-4764

New York, NY
Allan Inglis, Jr. MD
212-265-5566

Galesburg, IL
Dr. Myron Stachniw
309-342-0194

Springfield, IL
Dr. Gordon Allan
217-545-8865

Diagrams of Total Hip Replacement, Revision and Resurfacing technique taken from information at:
Http://www.swarminteractive.com/orthopedic/interactive/hip_total.ht
m
All diagrams and sketches were drawn by Peggathy Gabriel
All photographs taken by Dr. Kelly Coogan, DC
Art design on Cover by Peggathy Gabriel

Printed in the United Kingdom by
Lightning Source UK Ltd., Milton Keynes
140899UK00002B/73/A